Essential Reports in Paediatrics

Essential Reports in Paediatrics

C. MEADOWS
Specialist Registrar in Paediatrics
Royal United Hospital, NHS Trust
Bath, UK

N. HUMPHREYS
Specialist Registrar in Paediatrics
Royal United Hospital, NHS Trust
Bath, UK

A. BILLSON
Consultant Paediatrician
Royal United Hospital, NHS Trust
Bath, UK

© BIOS Scientific Publishers Limited, 2000

First published 2000

A CIP catalogue record for this book is available from the British Library.

ISBN 1 85996 168 1

BIOS Scientific Publishers Ltd
9 Newtec Place, Magdalen Road, Oxford OX4 1RE, UK
Tel. +44 (0)1865 726286. Fax +44 (0)1865 246823
World Wide Web home page: http://www.bios.co.uk/

Important Note from the Publisher
The information contained within this book was obtained by BIOS Scientific Publishers Ltd from sources believed by us to be reliable. However, while every effort has been made to ensure its accuracy, no responsibility for loss or injury whatsoever occasioned to any person acting or refraining from action as a result of information contained herein can be accepted by the authors or publishers.

The reader should remember that medicine is a constantly evolving science and while the authors and publishers have ensured that all dosages, applications and practices are based on current indications, there may be specific practices which differ between communities. You should always follow the guidelines laid down by the manufacturers of specific products and the relevant authorities in the country in which you are practising.

Production Editor: Paul Barlass.
Typeset by Creative Associates, Oxford, UK
Printed by The Cromwell Press, Trowbridge, UK

CONTENTS

CONTENTS

Dr Chris Alamenos, Specialist Registrar in Paediatrics, Taunton & Somerset Hospital, Musgrove Park, Taunton, Somerset TA1 5DA, UK

Dr Jo Brooks, Specialist Registrar in Paediatrics, Bath & West Community NHS Trust, Newbridge Hill, Bath BA1 3QE, UK

Dr Colin Downie, Staff Grade Paediatrician, Royal United Hospital NHS Trust, Combe Park, Bath BA1 3NG, UK

Dr Fiona Finlay, Consultant Community Paediatrician, Bath & West Community NHS Trust, Newbridge Hill, Bath BA1 3QE, UK

Dr Rosemary Jones, Senior Registrar in Paediatrics, Bath & West Community NHS Trust, Newbridge Hill, Bath BA1 3QE, UK

Dr Patricia May, Specialist Registrar in Paediatrics, Southampton General Hospital, Tremona Road, Southampton, Hants SO16 6YD, UK

Dr Alex Powell, Senior House Officer in Paediatrics, Bristol Hospital for Sick Children, St Michael's Hill, Bristol BS2 8BJ, UK

Dr David Olliffe, Specialist Registrar in Paediatrics, Northampton General Hospital, Billing Road, Northampton NN1 5BD, UK

Dr Miles Wagstaff, Specialist Registrar in Paediatrics, Great Ormond Street Hospital, Great Ormond Street, London WC1 3JH, UK

A&E	accident and emergency
ACPC	area child protection committee
ADH	additional duty hours
AIDS	acquired immune deficiency syndrome
ALTE	apparent life-threatening episode
APLS	advanced paediatric life support
BAPM	British Association of Perinatal Medicine
BCG	Bacillus de Calmette-Guérin
BPA	British Paediatric Association
BPSU	British Paediatric Surveillance Unit
CCST	certificate of completion of specialist training
CCTR	Cochrane controlled trials register
CDSR	Cochrane database of systematic reviews
CESDI	confidential enquiry into stillbirths and deaths in infancy
CFC	chlorofluorocarbon
CHIMP	Commission for Health Improvement
CHT	congenital hypothyroidism
CME	continuing medical education
CMO	clinical medical officer
CNS	central nervous system
CPAP	continuous positive airway pressure
CPD	continuing professional development
CRMD	Cochrane review methodology database
DARE	database of abstracts of reviews of effectiveness
DCCT	diabetes control and complications trial
DCH	diploma in child health
DHSS	Department of Health and Social Security
DKA	diabetic ketoacidosis
DMSA	dimercapto succinic acid
DoH	Department of Health
DTP	diphtheria, tetanus and pertussis (vaccine)
ECG	electrocardiography
ECME	external continuing medical education
EPO	emergency protection order
EU	European Union
FTTA	fixed-term training appointment
GMC	General Medical Council
GP	general practitioner
Hb	haemoglobin
HHV	human herpesvirus
HIB	*Haemophilus influenzae* type B
HIV	human immunodeficiency virus
ICME	internal continuing medical education
IDDM	insulin dependent diabetes mellitus
IgE	immunoglobulin E
JCVI	Joint Committee of Vaccination and Immunization
kPa	kilopascals

LAS	locum appointment for service
LAT	locum appointment for training
MCUG	micturating cystourethrogram
MDI	metered dose inhaler
MMR	measles, mumps and rubella (vaccine)
MRCP	Member of the Royal College of Physicians
MRCPCH	Member of the Royal College of Paediatrics and Child Health
NHS	National Health Service
NICE	National Institute of Clinical Excellence
NSF	national service framework
NSPCC	National Society for the Prevention of Cruelty to Children
NTN	national training number
$PaCO_2$	arterial carbon dioxide tension
PaO_2	arterial oxygen tension
PCG	Primary Care Group
PEF	peak expiratory flow
PHLS	Public Health Laboratory Service
PKU	phenylketonuria
QPC	Quality of Practice Committee
RCPCH	Royal College of Paediatrics and Child Health
RDS	respiratory disease syndrome
RITA	record of in-training assessment
RSV	respiratory syncytial virus
SaO_2	arterial oxygen saturation
SBNS	Society of British Neurological Surgeons
SCMO	senior clinical medical officer
SEN	special educational needs
SHO	senior house officer
SpR	Specialist Registrar
SSEN	statement of special educational needs
SSNS	steroid sensitive nephrotic syndrome
STA	Specialist Training Authority
UKCCSG	UK Children's Cancer Study Group
UKOS	UK oscillation study
UN	United Nations
UNICEF	United Nations International Children's Emergency Fund
USS	ultrasound scan
UTI	urinary tract infection
VSpR	visiting specialist registrar
VTN	visiting training number
VTS	vocational training scheme
VUR	vesicoureteric reflux
VZIG	varicella zoster immunoglobulin
WHO	World Health Organization

PREFACE

Every year sees the publication of a mountain of reports which have a direct bearing on the practice of paediatrics. It is difficult for an individual clinician to keep track of which reports they need to read. This book contains the key points and recommendations of 52 Working Party reports and other documents. A book of this kind can never be comprehensive but we have tried to highlight the documents with which the paediatrician should currently be familiar. The précised reports act as quick references to the key findings. However, the book is not intended to remove the need to read the original report and full references are given.

Documents summarized include important Government Acts, such as the Children Act 1989, and reports relating to Child Protection and the Development of Children's Services. There are sections on Child Health and Public Health, International Policy and Ethics, as well as Education, Training and Manpower. We have also included a section on Clinical Practice and Guidelines: this identifies reports which are consensus statements or include recommendations for good practice.

We are grateful to members of the department of Paediatrics at the Royal United Hospital, Bath and the Bath & West Community Child Health department who made suggestions as to which reports to include. Some of the reports were read and summarized by colleagues who presented them for discussion at our weekly Higher Professional training sessions. A list of those who contributed in this way is given on page viii.

We are also grateful to the Royal College of Paediatrics and Child Health for their help and support in the collation of this book, in particular their kind permission to reproduce verbatim the Duties of a Paediatrician (see page 1).

We have made every effort to accurately summarize the main points of each report. However, anyone planning to take decisions on the basis of a particular report or wishing to make direct quotes should refer to the original document.

We hope that this book will prove useful to paediatricians, both in training and career grade posts, and that there will be future editions and perhaps electronic updates.

Caroline Meadows
Nigel Humphreys
Amanda Billson

Duties of a Paediatrician

KEY POINTS
- Defines what is required of a Paediatrician
- Forms part of the Royal College of Paediatrics Oath
- Reproduced verbatim from the College handbook below

Paediatricians should commit themselves to practice in accordance with the Objects of the College and the UN Convention on the Rights of the Child.

Paediatricians have a responsibility to safeguard the reputation of paediatrics through their personal clinical practice and through participation in continuing professional development, enabling them to maintain and enhance their knowledge, skills and competence for effective clinical practice to meet the needs of children.

Paediatricians should recognize the limitations of their skills and seek advice and support when this would be in the best interests of the child.

Paediatricians should espouse paediatric research and promote interchange between medical science and clinical practice as it affects the life and health of children.

Paediatricians should pay due regard to the domestic, sociological, environmental and genetic dimensions of the health of children.

Paediatricians, whatever their specialty interest, should understand their particular responsibilities for the holistic and life-long health of children who come under their care: each contact is an opportunity for health promotion and disease prevention.

Paediatricians should serve as clinicians to the individual child while contributing to public health medicine.

Paediatricians should be aware of current medical and political affairs affecting the lives and health of children.

Paediatricians should serve as advocates for the health needs of children locally, nationally and internationally.

Paediatricians should see themselves as ambassadors for children and for the specialty of paediatrics.

Above all, paediatricians should be courteous and compassionate in all their dealings with children, their parents and other carers, placing the child's best interests at the centre of all clinical considerations.

REFERENCE

1. Duties of a Paediatrician. *Royal College of Paediatrics and Child Health Handbook 1999–2000*. London: Royal College of Paediatrics and Child Health; 1999. 25.

UK GOVERNMENT ACTS, POLICIES AND REPORTS

The Children Act 1989

KEY POINTS

- Welfare of the child is paramount
- The Welfare Checklist
- The 'No Order' principle
- Parental *Responsibilities* rather than *Rights*
- Legal position of unmarried fathers is changed
- Consent by older children is introduced
- Provides orders for the protection of children
- Regulation of children's homes
- Child minding regulations introduced

The Children Act 1989 [1] was introduced by the Department of Health (DoH) in 1989 as a wide ranging reform of the law as it relates to children.

The Act changed the way in which the law regards children. The courts now have to consider the welfare of the child as their prime consideration. In doing this, courts have to take into account a number of considerations, which together comprise the Welfare Checklist.

The Welfare Checklist includes:

- the wishes and feelings of the child (with regard to age and understanding);
- the child's needs (physical, emotional or educational);
- the effect upon the child of any order that may be placed;
- regard for the whole child (including age, gender, background, etc.);
- the harm which the child is likely to suffer.

Before putting any order in place the court has to be sure that doing so is better than not placing the order (the so called 'No Order' principle). Parental Responsibility is defined. Unmarried fathers are not given this responsibility as a right, though they can acquire it through the court or through an agreement with the mother.

The Act defines several orders to be used in child proceedings: a contact order, a prohibited steps order and a residence order for use in family proceedings. These orders act in the way their names imply. There is also a specific issue order which is used to determine a specific question that has arisen in respect of parental responsibility such as whether or not a child should receive a disputed treatment.

For paediatricians, Part V of the act is the most important as it deals with the protection of children. In particular, Section 44 defines the Emergency Protection Order (EPO), its powers and restrictions. The EPO replaces the place of safety order.

An EPO:

- may be applied for by the local authority, or an authorized person;
- lasts for up to 8 days, with the possibility of extension for a further 7 days;
- may only be placed if the court is satisfied that:

1. the child is likely to suffer significant harm if he is not removed;
2. enquiries are being made and these are being frustrated by lack of access to the child, which is urgently required;

- allows for restriction of access;
- allows for medical and/or psychiatric assessment of the child.

Other orders defined include a Child Assessment Order and an order allowing a police constable to remove a child to suitable accommodation or to prevent removal from such accommodation.

When any of the above child protection orders is put in place, the local authority then has a duty to investigate the circumstances of the order and to decide if further action is required. The local authority may request assistance from the local health authority, which has a duty to assist.

The concept of 'significant harm' is not an absolute, but rather depends upon examination of the child's health and development in comparison to a similar child.

Other parts of the Act define the obligations of local authorities to children and their families. Broadly they are required to 'safeguard and promote the welfare of children within their area who are in need' and crucially to 'promote the upbringing of such children by their families'. As part of this they must facilitate the work of others, including voluntary organizations, toward this aim.

Part IV deals with care, supervision and educational supervision orders. A Care Order requires the local authority to take the child into their care as long as the order remains in place. A Supervision Order requires the supervisor to 'advise, assist and befriend' the child. Education Supervision Orders are used when a child of compulsory school age is not being properly educated.

The remainder of the act deals with the regulation of community homes, voluntary homes, registered children's homes, private fostering and child minding.

The regulations on child minding allow the local authority to specify a limit on the number of children a child minder may care for. Childminders are required to keep records, including the name and address, of all children in their care. They must also keep records of any helpers they use, and any other persons living in the premises used. Provision is made for annual inspection of premises used for child minding.

REFERENCE

1. *The Children Act 1989*. The Stationary Office. 1989.

Education Act 1996

KEY POINTS

- Defines special educational needs
- Regulates the provision of education for children with special educational needs
- Imposes a statutory duty of assessment and provision on the local education authority
- Regulates the statement of special educational needs and its maintenance
- Aims to provide education for children with special educational needs within mainstream schools

Produced by Her Majesty's Government in 1996, the Education Act [1] regulates the provision of education in England and Wales. Part IV of the Act is of direct interest to paediatricians and provides for children with special educational needs (SENs).

A child is defined as having an SEN if they have a learning difficulty which results in the child needing special educational provision. A learning difficulty means that the child has 'significantly greater difficulty in learning than the majority of children of that age', or a disability which prevents or hinders the child from using normal school facilities.

An overriding principle of the Act is that, where possible, children with an SEN should be educated in mainstream schools. To enable this, schools are required to identify, and provide for, children with SEN.

The local education authority is responsible for arranging an assessment of educational needs for those children who may need special educational provision. Parents may also request an assessment. Once the decision to assess a child is taken, the parents must be informed and given a minimum of 29 days to respond. If as a result of the assessment it is decided that the child needs special educational provision, then the authority must make and maintain a statement of special educational need (SSEN). The SSEN should state the results of the assessment, and the provision required to meet the identified needs. The statement should also specify the type of school necessary to meet the child's needs. It may also name a specific school. Parents are given the right to appeal against the provision, or non-provision of an SSEN, or its contents. SSENs are required to be reviewed at least annually.

Special provision is made in the Act for the assessment of children under the age of 2 years. This may be done at the request of the parents and requires their consent. If a child under 5 years of age is thought to need assessment by a health authority or National Health Service (NHS) Trust, the parents must be informed that an assessment is thought necessary, and the local authority must be informed.

The Act makes provision for a Special Educational Needs Tribunal who hear appeals related to the provision for children with an SEN.

This part of the Act concludes by detailing the institutions in which the needs of children with an SEN may be met. Special schools must be approved by the Secretary of State. Independent schools may also be approved under this part of the Act.

REFERENCE

1. *The Education Act 1996*. The Stationary Office. 1996.

The Health of the Nation – A Strategy for England

KEY POINTS

- Aims to improve the health of the general population
- Aims to prevent avoidable ill health
- Sets targets for health improvements

The Health of the Nation is a White Paper introduced by the Conservative Government in 1992, with the aim of improving the health of the general population through the prevention of avoidable ill health [1]. It suggests targets for improvements in health, and proposes strategies for achieving these targets involving both disease prevention and health promotion, an approach previously used in the World Health Organization (WHO) document 'Health For All by the Year 2000' [2].

The White Paper uses the concepts of key areas, objectives and targets.

- Key areas are health issues identified as having the greatest scope or need for cost-efficient improvement. Each key area is a major cause of premature death or avoidable ill health, with available interventions offering a realistic chance of improvement.
- Objectives are set for each key area to improve health.
- Specific targets are then set for each key area, and these targets are monitored.

Although not immediately obvious, all of the key areas are relevant to the health of children, from birth to adolescence and beyond. In many ways, success with children, especially in the adoption of healthy lifestyles, is even more important. Many unhealthy lifestyles start in childhood or adolescence, whether it be poor diet, lack of exercise, smoking or sexual practices.

The specific key areas, objectives and targets of the Health of the Nation can be summarized as follows.

1. Coronary heart disease (CHD) and stroke
The targets set include a reduction in the rates of both CHD and stroke in both those under 65, and those between 65 and 74 years of age. This is to be achieved through health education encouraging a reduction in the known risk factors, namely:

- smoking;
- excess consumption of fat and salt;
- consumption of alcohol;
- lack of physical activity.

2. Cancers

The measures proposed centre around improving uptake of the national breast and cervical screening programmes, through promoting their values and by improving computerization.

Additionally, excessive exposure to sunlight is to be discouraged, and the rates of smoking reduced.

3. Mental illness

Specific targets are set for a reduction in suicide rates, as well as a general 'improvement in the health and social functioning' of the mentally ill. This is to be achieved by improving the services available to the mentally ill, as well as improving supervision. Staff are to be better trained, and good practice guidelines developed and adopted.

4. HIV, AIDS and sexual health

The targets are a reduction in the incidence of gonorrhoea as an indicator of human immunodeficiency virus (HIV) and acquired immune deficiency syndrome (AIDS) trends, and a decrease in the number of pregnancies in those under 16 years. These targets are to be achieved by public health campaigns aimed at drug misusers and school children, by improving treatment and support for those with HIV, and by making family planning services more comprehensive and more available.

5. Accidents

Many accidents are avoidable through health education, and other measures such as improved planning and design of the environment. This 'key area' is particularly important for children, where accidents are the most common cause of death in those over 1 year of age. The targets set are to be met by involving all those interested parties: national and local government, voluntary organizations, employers and employees, and parents. Paediatricians are in regular contact with families, and are in an ideal position to give advice on safety and accident prevention.

Since the 'Health of the Nation' paper was produced in 1992, there has been a change of Government, and priorities have changed. Few, if any, of the targets have yet been reached, but the legacies of the report remain:

- increased data collection from the NHS;
- research and development is still directed towards the 'key areas';
- reports are published regularly on the state of the nation's health.

REFERENCES

1. *The Health of the Nation – A Strategy for England.* The Stationary Office. 1992.
2. Tarimo E, Creese A, eds. *Achieving health for all by the year 2000.* World Health Organization.

The Patient's Charter – Services for Young People

KEY POINTS

- Defines the rights and expectations of a child within the NHS
- Includes sections on children who are healthy, sick, hospitalized or have special needs or are in local authority care
- Outlines who to contact and how to get help
- Defines the roles of different health care professionals

This is an information booklet published by the NHS as an addition to the Patient's Charter, aimed at children and their parents and carers [1]. It provides information on what a child's rights are, and what their expectations should be, with regards to health promotion, developmental assessments, health education, adolescent issues and hospital attendance. It also provides information on where and how to obtain help and advice for specific needs such as dentistry, vision testing and behavioural problems. The booklet is divided into sections on the healthy child, the sick child, the child with special needs and children looked after by the local authority. The following is a summary of the most important rights.

THE HEALTHY CHILD

- Your child has a right to his/her health records and these must be confidential.
- You can expect your health visitor to give you a record of your child's health for you to keep.
- You can expect your child to be immunized if you want.
- You can expect your child's development to be checked regularly if you wish.
- Your child can expect to be offered a health check by a school nurse or doctor in the first year of primary school.
- If your child has asthma you can expect him/her to have access to an inhaler at school.
- When your child reaches adolescence you can expect him/her to receive health education in school.
- Young people can expect to see their doctor in confidence.

THE SICK CHILD

- You and your child have the right to an explanation of any treatment proposed and to take part in discussions about any treatment and care.
- You can expect your child to be cared for at home whenever possible.
- You can expect appropriate help from the community nursing team and the loan of equipment when nursing your child at home.
- Your child has a right to continue education out of school if he/she cannot go because of illness.

THE CHILD IN HOSPITAL

- If you go to an accident and emergency (A&E) department you can expect your child to be seen and assessed immediately and for there to be a separate area specially for children.
- If your child is admitted you can expect to be given a bed within 2 h.
- When referred by a GP you can expect an outpatients appointment within 26 weeks.
- You can expect to be seen within 30 min of your outpatient appointment time.
- For non-urgent treatment, the maximum wait for admission is guaranteed to be no longer than 18 months.
- You can expect your child to be looked after on a children's ward under the supervision of a paediatric consultant.
- You can expect your child to have a named, qualified children's nurse responsible for his/her care.
- You can expect to be able to stay with your child in hospital if you wish.
- You can expect to be able to accompany your child to the anaesthetic room and stay with him/her until he/she goes to sleep.
- You can expect all the staff you meet to wear name badges.
- Your child has a right to receive suitable education if in hospital for a long time.
- You can expect the hospital to tell your general practitioner (GP) when your child leaves hospital.

THE CHILD WITH SPECIAL NEEDS

This section does not list expectations and rights, but gives a brief outline of the statementing procedure (see also pages 6–7) and the type of professionals who may be involved in the care of a child with special needs.

THE CHILD LOOKED AFTER BY A LOCAL AUTHORITY

Local authority social services departments are expected to act as good parents to children in their care, to make a plan for the care of a child while away from home and to make every effort to arrange for a medical examination and written assessment before a child is placed away from home.

The final few pages of the booklet explains how patients may make a complaint about hospital services, social services or educational provision.

REFERENCE

1. NHS: *The Patient's Charter: Services for Children and Young People*. Department of Health. 1996.

A First Class Service: Quality in the New NHS

KEY POINTS

- Ten year modernization programme for the NHS to create 'the new NHS'
- Priority given to providing high quality, prompt service to all patients
- Clinical Governance is key and requires formal CPD programmes
- Abolition of the internal NHS market
- Introduction of NICE which will issue evidence-based clinical guidelines
- Introduction of NSFs to set service provision and organization standards
- Introduction of CHIMP to monitor quality and standards locally

This is a consultation document which sets out a 10-year agenda for modernizing the structure of the NHS with the aim of 'improving quality standards, efficiency, openness and accountability' [1]. The consultation period ended in September 1998 with the subsequent publication of this document later in the year by the Labour Government. Implementation of these changes began in 1999 with the setting up of a National Institute of Clinical Excellence (NICE).

The document praises the NHS and its work since it was set up but points out the need for radical changes to meet the current demands of society – aiming to prioritize giving high quality, prompt services to all patients. There are currently many inequalities in service provision ranging from drug availability to operation waiting times, and high variability in clinical practice and outcomes. The consultation document states these inequalities stem from four main causes: the internal NHS market, lack of clear national standards of care, lack of coherent assessment of which treatments work best and for who and, finally, lack of public accountability. Each of these areas has been targeted for change.

The internal NHS market will be abolished.

Quicker access to medical advice will result from cutting hospital waiting lists and introducing 24 h telephone advice lines nationwide – NHS Direct.

Clear national standards of service provision will be supported by evidence-based guidance, thus raising the quality of the NHS. There is recognition that local areas vary in their needs and the individual clinician will retain the power to make clinical decisions for individual patients. The national standards will be set through National Service Frameworks (NSFs) and through NICE. Responsibility for delivery will remain local and will require consistent monitoring arrangements and will result in increased accountability.

NICE will aim to provide evidence based medical guidance for clinicians – looking at drugs, devices, new and existing treatments and management of certain conditions, with regard to cost-effectiveness and clinical effectiveness. In the future there may be scope for NICE to look at public health issues such as screening. In addition, the established National Confidential Enquiries (e.g. Confidential Enquiry into Stillbirths and Deaths in Infancy (CESDI) [2]) will also come under the remit of NICE, hopefully giving power to their findings and influencing standard setting. This will help to ensure effective local clinical governance. Guidelines issued by NICE will be expected to be implemented across the NHS and there will be increasing challenges to local deviations from these guidelines. Information published by NICE will be available on the Internet (and possibly digital TV) and therefore available to the public, patients and all medical personnel.

The NSF will set standards of service provision and organization, with the aim of giving greater consistency in the availability and quality of services provided. Standards set will be evidence-based and will look at major care areas and disease groups, usually looking at one or two main areas each year. Areas chosen will include those where health inequalities are greatest or of most relevance, and areas of public concern. On a more local scale, NSFs will also put into place programmes to aid implementation of the guidelines produced by NICE. This may require further research and development projects, benchmarking and staff education. In addition it will create performance measures against which progress will be measured and hospitals can be compared to each other. The programme will start with mental health and coronary heart disease.

The standards will be delivered locally by a new system of clinical governance, continuing professional development and professional self-regulation. Monitoring of the standards will be done in three ways.

1. A Commission for Health Improvement (CHIMP): reviewing trusts and investigating when things go wrong.
2. A National Framework for Assessing Performance: seeing whether services meet quality objectives.
3. An annual National Survey of Patient and User Experience of the NHS: to see if services are meeting patients needs locally.

The CHIMP will be set up to monitor local service quality and to put this information in the public domain. To begin with it will be funded centrally, but eventually some of this may become local. The Commission will support local quality improvement development and perform 'spot checks' on new arrangements. Each trust will be examined every 3–4 years. Where there are problems that cannot be resolved locally, the Commission will intervene under the direction of the Secretary of State, or by invitation from trusts and health authorities. The Commission will investigate, recommend action to the Secretary of State and even have the power to remove executive directors and NHS Trust Chairs. Although involved in management issues, the main area of activity for the Commission will be clinical issues. In the future the Commission may also oversee and assist with external incident inquiries.

NICE and NSFs will set high standards. To make these effective will require a new system of clinical governance to monitor health care at a local level. Clinical governance is a 'framework through which NHS organizations are accountable for continuously improving the quality of their services and safeguarding high standards of care by creating an environment in which excellence in clinical care will flourish'. This will require lifelong learning for staff, professional self-regulation and external monitoring. There will be a national audit programme requiring the participation of all hospital doctors in their relevant specialties. National comparative audits will allow comparison of one doctor's performance against a national average. There will be policies aimed at identifying and remedying poor staff performance. Staff will be supported in expressing concerns about their colleagues' professional conduct and performance. There will also be clear policies regarding risk management. Where standards fall short of expectations urgent action will be taken to remedy this. Where necessary, the General Medical Council (GMC) will be involved. The Chief Executives will have ultimate responsibility for service quality in their trusts and will have to publish annual reports on quality assurance within their trust.

The report makes the point that the majority of health care is given outside hospital by primary health care teams. Primary care groups will also be expected to demonstrate a systematic approach to monitoring and developing clinical standards in the development of clinical governance. This will allow the development of primary care trusts. They will be supported by individual health authorities. The Royal College of General Practitioners will play an important role in supporting quality improvement by, for example, assessing performance before allowing membership.

The report goes on to highlight the importance of continuing professional development (CPD) [3] and lifelong learning as an investment in the future quality of the NHS. It suggests a more integrated approach to this, encompassing links between audit, clinical effectiveness and research and development. It recognizes that CPD programmes should be managed locally in order to meet local requirements. CPD should be instigated by first assessing the needs of an individual and/or organization, creating a personal development plan, implementing the plan, evaluating its effectiveness in terms of CPD intervention and patient care and then going back to the assessment stage in a perpetual cycle. The document states that the majority of health professionals should have training and development plans in place by April 2000.

Self-regulation will be another way of ensuring quality. This allows health professionals to set their own standards of professional service, conduct and discipline. Obviously this leaves professional bodies open to criticism and they must therefore be accountable for the standards they set and the way they enforce them. This should help boost public confidence.

Finally, the document lays out a framework for the changes detailed with anticipated dates for implementation running from 1998–2000.

REFERENCES

1. *A First Class Service: Quality in the new NHS*. Department of Health. 1998.
2. *Confidential Enquiry into Stillbirths and Deaths in Infancy*. 6th Annual Report. Maternal and Child Health Research Consortium. 1999.
3. *Continuing Medical Education*. London: Royal College of Paediatrics and Child Health. 1997.

The Ionizing Radiations Regulations Act 1985 & 1988

KEY POINTS
- The 1985 regulations aim to minimize radiation exposure of employees
- The 1988 regulations aim to minimize exposure of patients to radiation
- Only people with adequate training can carry out medical exposure to radiation
- People clinically directing the exposure are responsible for ensuring the procedure is carried out according to accepted standards
- Proof of training is required
- Requesting an X-ray is not the same as clinically directing the procedure

These legal regulations were introduced by the Government and are enforceable under the Health and Safety at Work Act 1974. They set out the basic safety standards for the protection of workers, the general public and patients against the risks from ionizing radiation [1,2].

The 1985 regulations aim to minimize the exposure of employees and the public. Amongst other things they define dose limits, deal with the designation of controlled/supervised areas and the designation of classified workers.

The 1988 regulations deal with the protection of persons undergoing medical examination and treatment. Only people with adequate training can carry out exposures to radiation. A core of knowledge is outlined which is required by people clinically or physically directing the exposure. Proof of training in the form of a certificate from an appropriate body is required. Definitions of clinically and physically directing are given.

Clinically directing
For all exposures to radiation there should be someone responsible for clinically directing the exposure. They are responsible for ensuring that it is carried out according to accepted standards. This person is usually a consultant radiologist/radiotherapist, but may be cardiologists carrying out catheterization or a paediatrician screening for a capsule in a small bowel biopsy. Staff requesting an X-ray are asking for a clinical opinion from a radiologist and not clinically directing.

Physically directing
This is the person who presses the exposure button or injects the isotope. It is usually a radiographer. They should select the necessary procedures to minimize the dose to the patient as far as it is reasonably practical. Employers also have a responsibility to ensure that records relating to radiation equipment are kept, that an expert in the application of physics is available and that employees are suitably trained.

REFERENCES

1. *Ionizing Radiations Regulation Act 1985*. The Stationary Office. 1985.
2. *Ionizing Radiations Regulation Act 1988*. The Stationary Office. 1988.

The Welfare of Children in Hospital (The Platt Report)

KEY POINTS

- Separate inpatient and outpatient facilities for adults and children
- Pre-admission preparations including a hospital visit and leaflet
- Qualified sick children's nurses on each paediatric nursing team
- Open visiting for parents
- Parents allowed to stay with children under 5 years of age
- Indoor and outdoor play areas
- Children in hospital should have access to education
- Minimize distress associated with medical intervention
- Special facilities for children with special needs

This report was written in 1958 under the chairmanship of Sir Harry Platt, former president of the Royal College of Surgeons [1]. The Central Health Services Council appointed the committee in 1956 with a brief to make a special study of the arrangements made in hospitals for the welfare of children and to make recommendations to hospital authorities. The report is made up of four main sections, dealing with preparation for admission, admission procedure, in-patient care and discharge, respectively. The publication of this report fundamentally changed the way children were treated in hospital.

The emotional effects of hospitalizing children can be life-long, not only because of the procedures they undergo, but also because of the effects of separation from their families. Therefore, every effort should be made to avoid admission, and to meet the specialist needs of the child at home.

The main recommendations are as poignant today as they were in 1958 and it is for this reason that we have included this report. Many of the recommendations form part of the Patient's Charter (see also pages 10 and 11). The recommendations are listed below.

1. Hospitals should have a separate children's outpatient department or a separate waiting room in an adult department or casualty department. Children and adolescents should not be nursed on an adult ward. There should be facilities for inside and outside play. Each nursing team should include a sick children's nurse and the child should have access to other staff such as a social worker, occupational therapist and nursery nurses.
2. Prior to admission there should be hospital open days allowing families to have preparatory talks with hospital staff. Hospital leaflets and letters should be available. GPs and health visitors should give explanations and reassurance to children and families.
3. Whilst in hospital children should be allowed to keep their personal possessions and wear their own clothes. Children should have access to education. Admission of mothers should be considered in the first few days for children under 5 years of

age. There should be unrestricted visiting from parents ('at any reasonable hour of the day'). There should be facilities for visitors such as a playroom for siblings and a canteen. Parents should be kept informed of their child's progress by both nursing and medical staff. There should be ward prayers and Sunday school.

4. Unpleasant medical techniques should be kept to a minimum. An explanation of unpleasant techniques should be given to children. There should be separate treatment and recovery rooms so other children do not witness distressing procedures. Parents should be present at recovery from anaesthesia. There should be limited discussions between medical staff in front of children.

5. Children with special needs may need more in the way of pre-admission preparation. They should have access to any special equipment that is necessary. They should be taught by teachers who have specialist skills or can access such expertise.

6. On discharge from hospital, parents should be warned about behavioural problems that may arise at home, and how to get advice on how to deal with them. General practitioners should be informed in advance and sent as full a report as possible.

7. Doctors, nurses and other staff who care for children should be given training about the emotional needs of children in hospital, and how to adjust their procedures to suit children.

REFERENCE

1. Report of the Central Health Services Council Committee. *The Welfare of Children in Hospital (The Platt Report)*. The Stationary Office. 1958.

CHILD HEALTH AND PUBLIC HEALTH

Health for all Children – The Hall Report

KEY POINTS
- Basis of child health promotion in UK
- Emphasizes primary prevention
- Retains the core programme of child health surveillance
- Clear referral guidelines
- Targeted health services
- Importance of personal child health record emphasized

Produced by the Third Joint Working Party of Child Health Surveillance in 1996, this report forms the basis of current child health surveillance practice in the UK [1].

The report marked a change in emphasis away from screening (secondary prevention) towards primary prevention. It introduced the term 'child health promotion' encompassing both the older term, 'child health surveillance', and primary prevention. The Child Health Promotion Programme is developed as a series of key recommendations. Alongside these recommendations are many suggestions for the audit of clinical practice.

The core programme of immunizations and reviews previously in place is retained. This core surveillance programme consists of:

- the neonatal examination, either in hospital or by the GP;
- contact by the health visitor in the first 2 weeks;
- the 6-week check, by the GP;
- immunizations at 2, 3 and 4 months (DTP + HIB);
- a check between 6 and 9 months, by the health visitor or GP;
- MMR vaccination at 13 months;
- review by the health visitor between 18 and 24 months;
- pre-school check by a GP.

At each stage there are suggestions for appropriate health education topics for discussion with the parents by the health professional.

The report discusses child health promotion looking at the assessment of need, targeting of support and the effects of environment.

Looking at primary prevention the report reviews:

1. Immunizations and the prevention of infectious disease, where the emphasis is on increasing the uptake of immunizations. Other issues are addressed including basic food hygiene and personal hygiene education.
2. Sudden infant death syndrome, the major risk factors and approaches to reducing its incidence, including reducing parental smoking.
3. Prevention of unintentional injury.

4. Nutrition and, specifically, the benefits of breast feeding as part of a baby-friendly initiative. The report also summarizes current thinking on vitamin K prophylaxis and emphasizes the need to ensure that, if oral doses are used, subsequent doses are given.
5. Dental and oral disease and its prevention.

Secondary prevention (detection of latent disease) is examined and the role of screening is discussed. The benefits of early detection are examined in some detail, concluding that in many cases it is advantageous. The criteria for a screening programme are examined, including Wilson and Jungner's criteria [2]. The potential for litigation as a result of 'missed' diagnoses in screening is also addressed, suggesting that unreliable screening tests are open to litigation.

Examination in the context of screening is discussed, with procedures for congenital hip dislocation, congenital heart disease, hypertension, asthma and undescended testes presented in some detail.

The monitoring of growth is given extensive coverage and recommendations are made emphasizing the importance of growth monitoring in paediatric practice.

The report concludes by summarizing the 1996 Child Health Promotion Programme, giving details of the core surveillance programme. Since the publication of this report there have been a number of changes to the core programme including the introduction of the meningitis C vaccination(s).

REFERENCES

1. Hall MB. (ed). *Health for All Children. Report of the Third Joint Working Party on Child Health Surveillace*. 3rd edn. Oxford: Oxford University Press, 1996.
2. Wilson JMG, Jungner G. *Principles and practice of screening for disease. Public Health Papers No. 34*. Geneva: World Health Organization. 1968.

Inequalities in Health (The Black Report)

KEY POINTS

- Identifies inequalities in health between social classes
- Increased child mortality rates in children of unskilled workers vs. professionals
- Increased death rates in unskilled workers vs. professionals
- Makes recommendations to try to reduce these inequalities

This landmark report [1] underlies many subsequent reports, policies and enquiries. It was commissioned by the Secretary of State in 1977 and compiled by a working party headed by Sir Douglas Black. The working party's objectives were to identify inequalities in health between the social classes and to identify factors that might influence health. From this they were to draw implications for policy and further research.

FINDINGS

- Increased mortality rate of children born to unskilled workers compared to professionals.
- Increased death rate in both sexes and at all ages in unskilled workers compared to professionals.
- Increased chronic illness in both sexes of unskilled group compared to professional groups.
- Severe under-utilization of health services, especially preventative services, by working class groups compared to professional group.
- Increased number of accidents in children of unskilled workers compared to professionals.

RECOMMENDATIONS

- Measures to improve health and welfare of mothers and children (e.g. improved access to antenatal care, provision of pre-school nurseries, improved maternal and child benefits).
- More community resources to promote home care of elderly and disabled.
- Institution of screening programmes, e.g. for hypertension.
- Establishment of health promotion programmes and national goals to improve diet, increase exercise, and reduce smoking and drinking.
- Adequate provision of education, housing and social services support to those in need.
- Establishment of a Health Development Council to advise and plan national policy to reduce inequalities in health.

OUTCOME

In a review 7 years later, it was noted that most recommendations had been rejected, and there had been a lack of action, particularly at the national level.

Locally, however:

• some health and social service projects have led to improved access for deprived communities to primary health care;
• awareness has been raised, and health databases compiled;
• there have been initiatives by employers to highlight health promotion and disease prevention in the workplace.

The reduction of health inequalities between social groups is one of the targets of the WHO 'Health for All by the Year 2000' [2] and this has been embraced by the UK government.

REFERENCES

1. *Inequalities in Health: Report of a Research Working Group (The Black Report)*. HMSO. 1998.
2. Tarimo E, Creese A, eds. *Achieving health for all by the year 2000*. Geneva: World Health Organization.

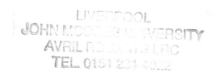

Confidential Enquiry into Stillbirths and Deaths in Infancy

KEY POINTS

- Annual report into deaths of foetuses from 20 weeks gestation to infants up to 1 year of age
- Aims to make recommendations to reduce mortality in these groups

The Confidential Enquiry into Stillbirths and Deaths in Infancy (CESDI) [1] is a National enquiry initiated by the DoH in 1992 to look at all late foetal, neonatal and infant deaths. Its aim is to reduce mortality in these groups. Its results are collated and published on an annual basis. Since April 1999, responsibility for CESDI has lain with the NICE. Data is collected via the Rapid Report Form which should be filled in by the relevant medical practitioner following death of a foetus or infant from 20 weeks gestation to 1 year of age.

The report has two components:

- a survey of all deaths from 20 weeks gestation to 1 year after birth;
- a confidential enquiry into some of these deaths by a multidisciplinary panel who assess the circumstances of death and care given to individual babies, with the aim of highlighting ways in which the death could have been avoided; such as ways to reduce the number of sudden infant deaths [2].

Each year different aspects of care are focused on. Statistics are given for the UK as a whole but shorter, regional reports are also available.

SIXTH ANNUAL REPORT 1996–1997

Findings

- In 1997, 10 418 deaths notified: 1299 legal abortions, 1774 late foetal deaths, 3440 stillbirths, 2648 neonatal deaths, 1257 post-neonatal deaths. The stillbirth rate is significantly less for the first time since 1993. Other rates are unchanged.
- The '1 in 10' Enquiry looked at 537 deaths from 24 weeks gestation to 27 days of life, where birth weight was over 1 kg and there were no major congenital abnormalities. Half of the stillbirths and 72% of intrapartum deaths were found to have received suboptimal care, where different care might or would reasonably have been expected to have made a difference. They recommend the need to review standards of antenatal and intrapartum care.
- The '4 kg and over' enquiries looked at 151 deaths in babies with birth weight over 4 kg and aged under 28 days. Three per cent were born to mothers with pre-existing diabetes mellitus and 8% with gestational diabetes. They recommend better supervision and early use of insulin in hyperglycaemic women, letting the delivery team know when a large baby is suspected clinically so that they can be alert for

delay in labour, the possibility of shoulder dystocia and ensure the presence of experienced staff to supervise any instrumental delivery. They also highlight the need for delivery suites to have clear protocols for calling a paediatrician who has adequate experience in resuscitation skills. They should be aware of the possible consequences of difficult deliveries and the possibility of pneumothorax in a baby not responding to resuscitation.
- Perinatal pathology: a review of post-mortem reports concludes that there is still great variability in the standard to which these are done and that skills need to be improved. CESDI are aware that obtaining informed consent for post-mortem examination is difficult and have published leaflets for parents. They have also produced a leaflet entitled 'The Foetal and Infant Post-mortem, brief notes for the Professional' which covers legal requirements, consent and information about the procedure itself.
- Record keeping was found to be poor in one-third of cases reviewed, with the main problem being failure to document events adequately.

Some of the topics covered in previous reports are listed below.

Fifth annual report
Sudden unexpected deaths in infancy: the explained group, Antepartum term stillbirths, Place of delivery, Ruptured uterus, Shoulder dystocia.

Fourth annual report
Intrapartum related deaths.

Third annual report
Sudden unexpected deaths in infancy: following which these key recommendations [2] were issued:

- "Back to sleep": babies should lie supine for sleeping and not prone;
- "Feet to foot"/head uncovered: babies should be placed at the foot of the cot so they cannot slide down under the covers;
- not too hot;
- smoke free zone;
- prompt medical advice;
- bed sharing for comfort not for sleep.

REFERENCES
1. *Confidential Enquiry into Stillbirths and Deaths in Infancy.* 6th Annual Report. London: Maternal and Child Health Research Consortium. 1999.
2. *Reduce the risk of cot death: an easy guide.* Department of Health free leaflet, revised February 2000. Available on tel: 0800 555777; www.doh.gov.uk/cot death/

CHILD PROTECTION

Child Protection – Messages from Research

KEY POINTS

- Clear definitions are needed when dealing with child abuse
- Many children are neglected and this causes significant harm
- Child protection investigations should aim to support families of children in need
- About a quarter of abused children are re-abused
- Professionals should be sensitive, have a wide perspective on child abuse and have determination to enhance the quality of children's lives

This report was produced in 1995 by the Dartington Social Research Unit [1]. Several high profile cases had raised public awareness of the issues of child protection and concerns about the safety of children. Questions were raised about decision making, the nature of intervention and the provision of services by different agencies. As a result of these questions and concerns, the UK Government commissioned 20 individual research projects and the key messages from these are outlined in this report. The overall aim of the report is 'to inform everyone working in the child protection field and ultimately to enhance the welfare of the child'.

The report starts with an overview and then summarizes the individual research reports.

The overview is divided into four main sections:

1. **The problems of definition.** It is suggested that many children live in environments where their health and development are neglected and it is the corrosiveness of long-term maltreatment that causes psychological impairment or significant harm. Professionals need clear parameters in order to act with confidence to protect vulnerable children.
2. **The child protection process.** Against a background of 350 000 children being in low warmth, high criticism environments and who are likely to suffer if their families are not helped, it is suggested that child protection investigators should both investigate maltreatment and evaluate how a family could benefit from support. Approximately 160 000 children are referred annually to the child protection process, with 40 000 being the subject of a child protection conference. As 96% of children remain at home and the majority of those who are separated are swiftly reunited, it is important to involve the family and the child in the child protection process, working in partnership with professionals.
3. **How effective is the child protection process?** The difficulty in measuring outcomes is discussed. Studies show that about a quarter of children are re-abused and an Oxford study on sexual abuse defined 43% of the cases investigated as 'unsafe' 9 months later. It is acknowledged that 'a suspicion of child abuse has

traumatic effects on families. Good professional practice can ease parents' anxiety and lead to cooperation that helps protect the child'.

4. **How can professionals best protect children?** Five pre-conditions of effective practice to protect children and promote their welfare are described:
   1. sensitive and informed professional/client relationships;
   2. an appropriate balance of power between key parties;
   3. a wide perspective on child abuse;
   4. effective supervision and training of social workers;
   5. a determination to enhance the quality of children's lives.

The second half of the report gives clear individual summaries of each research project with a note made of points of interest. Studies include:

- the prevalence of child sexual abuse in Britain;
- professional intervention in child sexual abuse;
- normal family sexuality and sexual knowledge in children;
- parental control within the family;
- paternalism or partnership? Family involvement in the child protection process;
- parental perspectives in cases of suspected child abuse.

At the end of the book there are 12 exercises which may be used in single agency or multidisciplinary training. They are scenarios aimed at stimulating discussion about child abuse, for example 'discuss the issue of a 3-year-old who clings to the health visitor during a home visit and is reluctant to return to her mother'.

REFERENCE

1. Report of the Dartington Social Research Unit. *Child Protection - Messages From Research*. The Stationary Office. 1995.

Report of the Enquiry into Child Abuse in Cleveland 1987

KEY POINTS

- An enquiry into the unprecedented rise in the diagnosis of child sexual abuse in Cleveland during 1987
- Highlighted the misinterpretation of reflex anal dilatation as a sign of child sexual abuse
- Found poor interdisciplinary communication
- Made recommendations regarding examining children
- Recommended a review of training arrangements in child abuse

There was an unprecedented rise in the diagnosis of child sexual abuse in Cleveland mainly during May and June 1987. An enquiry was set up, led by Lord Justice Elizabeth Butler-Sloss. Its terms of reference were 'to examine the arrangements for dealing with suspected cases of child abuse in Cleveland since January 1, 1987, including, in particular, cases of child sex abuse, and to make recommendations'. The results of this enquiry, published in 1987, are now commonly known as The Cleveland Report and have changed the way child sex abuse is approached [1].

On January 1, 1987, a new doctor started work in Cleveland. She had previously worked in another area where she had seen two children with the 'reflex relaxation and anal dilatation' sign which a colleague had suggested was found in children subjected to anal sexual abuse. This colleague later became involved in the diagnosis of some of the cases. On the basis of this sign, the new doctor made many diagnoses of sexual abuse in children, resulting in several arrests and the placement of many children in care. Some of the cases were in children with constipation and some in children who had made no complaints of abuse. The signs persisted even in some children taken away into care and a police surgeon, supported by another doctor, challenged the diagnosis of sexual abuse. Their challenge was discounted.

Many of the older children diagnosed as having been abused were interviewed by police, without the presence of social workers.

By the first week of May 1987, 23 children had been diagnosed as having suffered sexual abuse and a crisis meeting was held with social workers. At this time the police were concerned that the social service guidelines excluded police surgeons from the diagnostic procedures. The police surgeons felt the doctor's diagnoses were suspect.

In June 1987, many further diagnoses of child sexual abuse were made and on one evening 11 place of safety orders were applied for. The MP Stuart Bell was informed of the situation and met the parents support group which had formed. The clerk of the justices was also anxious about the large number of cases and the fact that the doctors were asking for parental access to be denied. On the same day the doctors were asked to meet Professor Sir Bernard Tomlinson, Chairman of the Northern Region. Complaints were presented, but the panel could 'find no reason to recommend their suspension from duties'. A regional reference group was set up to provide a second opinion in certain cases and some parents also arranged their own second opinion. Later in the month the MP gave the Minister for Health a dossier of cases he had investigated and as a result a statutory enquiry was announced.

The Cleveland report concluded that initial 'possible suspicions' were gradually changed to 'unequivocal diagnoses' in relation to the signs seen, particularly reflex anal dilatation. Although the second doctor involved had originally given support to the diagnoses, she later advised caution but this was ignored. A new Child Abuse Consultant had supported the diagnoses and her response dominated the thinking of the whole social services department. Wider assessments had been stopped, partly due to the large number of referrals. The police surgeon was described as being confrontational and because of this, his views were ignored. There was little inter-agency communication. Of the 121 children originally diagnosed by the two doctors as having been abused, only 23 had not returned home by the time of the report.

The report made many recommendations regarding the investigation of possible child abuse. Children's wishes and feelings should always be taken into account. Children should not be subjected to repeated examinations or interviews. Examinations should take place in a suitable and sensitive environment and be performed by suitably trained staff. Parents should be treated courteously, be kept well informed at every stage and be given written explanations of important decisions or orders. They should be invited to case conferences wherever possible. Where there are conflicting opinions, these must be put to the whole conference by medical witnesses. Social Services should seek orders for minimum periods of time, develop a code of practice and allow parental access where possible. The report recommended that the medical profession should agree on signs of sexual abuse and a consistent vocabulary to describe them. They should also ensure that appropriate forensic examination takes place, prepare accurate medical records, and seek informed consent. Where practitioners disagree in their findings they should try to resolve their differences and recognise that their purpose is to act in the best interests of the child.

The report recommended that area review committees should review training arrangements and establish specialist multidisciplinary assessment teams including an appropriate medical practitioner, a senior social worker and a suitable police officer.

REFERENCE

1. Butler-Sloss E. *Report of the Enquiry into Child Abuse in Cleveland 1987*. The Stationary Office. 1988.

FURTHER READING

1. *Child Sex Abuse – The Way Forward*. National Children's Bureau. 1988.
2. *Post Cleveland – The Implications for Training*. National Children's Bureau Training Advisory Group on Sexual Abuse of Children. London: Training Advisory Group on Sexual Abuse of Children. (See pages 34–35)
3. *Working Together – A Guide to Inter-agency Co-operation for the Protection of Children from Abuse*. HMSO. 1988. (now superseded by: *Working Together to Safeguard Children. A Guide to Inter-agency Working to Safeguard and Promote the Welfare of Children*. The Stationary Office. 1999.)

Post Cleveland – The Implications for Training

KEY POINTS

- Training recommendations for those involved in child protection – issued following the 1987 Cleveland Report
- Local responsibility of Area Child Protection Committees (ACPCs) to ensure adequate training of those involved in child protection
- Three levels of post-basic training with specific knowledge criteria for specific professionals

This document was published jointly by the National Children's Bureau and the Training Advisory Group on Sexual Abuse of Children [1]. It followed the outcry surrounding the Cleveland Report which found that children were wrongly being diagnosed as having been sexually abused, and that this problem was compounded by a lack of inter-agency cooperation.

The document sets out a recommended framework for training professionals who deal with cases of suspected child abuse. It emphasizes the importance of respecting the autonomy of children and the need for inter-agency cooperation.

Local area child protection committees will take responsibility for ensuring adequate provision of training and for setting standards in child abuse practice. This training needs to be monitored and regularly reviewed.

Individual training needs should be clearly identified so that the appropriate courses can be completed. Three levels of training course are proposed which are preceded by a basic qualifying course and an induction course.

Level 1
Post-basic training for all staff in direct contact with children and their families. It includes elementary child care law and question of consent, recognition and definition of child abuse and local procedure.

Level 2
Professional general training for staff with direct contact with children, with child care or management responsibilities. Alternatively, training for professionals who need specific skills such as paediatricians requiring training in forensic clinical examination. This level should include more detailed information about child sex abuse and law, counselling skills for peers and juniors, review of forensic issues and giving evidence in court.

For paediatricians it is recommended that they should be familiar with techniques for the examination of normal genitalia and their normal and pathological variants. They should also be able to identify social and emotional indicators of child sex abuse, and to recognize non-accidental and sexually significant injury. In addition, they should be familiar with the collection of forensic evidence and with examination for sexually transmitted disease. Paediatricians should be aware of the importance of the growth chart in identifying children at risk.

Recommendations are also made for the knowledge required by GPs, police surgeons, gynaecologists, psychiatrists, teachers, etc.

Level 3
Intensive training for professionals involved as consultants or in the provision of investigative or intervention programmes.

REFERENCE

1. *Post Cleveland - The Implications for Training*. National Children's Bureau Training Advisory Group on Sexual Abuse of Children. London: Training Advisory Group on Sexual Abuse of Children.

FURTHER READING

1. Butler-Sloss E. *Report of the Inquiry into Child Abuse in Cleveland 1987*. The Stationary Office. 1988. (see also pages 32–34).
2. *Working Together. A Guide to Arrangements for Inter-Agency Co-operation for the Protection of Children from Abuse*. The Stationary Office. 1988.
3. *Working Together to Safeguard Children*. Department of Health. The Stationary Office. 1999. (see also pages 37–39).

Working Together to Safeguard Children

KEY POINTS

- Replaces 'Working Together Under The Children Act'
- Outlines the roles of the agencies involved in child protection
- Provides guidance for the operation of child protection procedures
- Guides the operation of Area Child Protection Committees (ACPCs)

Produced in 1999, this document [1] replaces the older document 'Working Together Under The Children Act'. Its purpose is to provide an outline of the ways in which the multiple agencies involved in child protection should work together to protect children from abuse and neglect. It does not provide detailed information but rather presents a framework for detailed local implementation.

Abuse and neglect is discussed and the categories of abuse for the purpose of legislation are defined.

- Physical: acts directly or indirectly (as in Munchausen by proxy) causing physical harm.
- Emotional: acts or omissions which adversely affect a child's emotional development or well being.
- Sexual: acts in which the child is encouraged, or forced, to participate in sexual activities, or to observe them.
- Neglect: the persistent failure to meet the child's physical (i.e. food, shelter, protection from harm) or psychological needs.

Central to child abuse legislation is the concept of 'significant harm'. There is no absolute measure of this, but rather each case needs to be judged individually, looking at the full circumstances of the child. A relatively minor physical act might be judged as significant when observed in a child who is otherwise neglected.

Enabling the child to remain safely within his or her family, where possible is central to the Children Act (see pages 4–5). The report examines the stresses (such as poverty, drug abuse and mental illness) which act upon families and may impair children's development.

The report stresses that in child protection the focus of the involved professionals should be upon the child rather than the child protection process itself. The roles of the agencies involved in child protection (local authorities, social services, education services, health services, the police, etc.) are examined individually, setting each within the context of the others.

The role of health professionals includes recognizing children in need, cooperating with other agencies involved in child protection, and meeting the health needs of children and their families. Health services include the health authority, hospitals and community health services, primary care groups and trusts, GPs and other members of the multidisciplinary team.

The health authority sets the overall strategy for child protection. It should assist in planning services for children in need and their families and set standards for safeguarding children in the services it commissions. It should also identify the lead health professionals (paediatrician and nurse) who are responsible for health provision for child protection.

Hospital trusts and community health services provide acute and community services for children and their families. Each trust should also identify lead professionals for child protection. Trusts should ensure that all professionals coming into contact with children are aware of child protection issues and know how to involve the child protection team. Specialist paediatric advice should be available to non paediatricians treating children, such as A&E departments.

Primary Care Groups (PCGs) are a new addition to the NHS. They comprise groups of GP practices who will commission hospital and community health services (replacing GP fund holders). Some PCGs will become independent trusts (Primary Care Trusts). These trusts may themselves provide some community paediatric services, previously provided by Community Paediatric Trusts.

GPs and members of the Primary Health Care Team should be alert to children who are potentially in need. All members of the team need to be aware of, and have available a copy of, the local Area Child Protection Procedures.

Each local authority should have an Area Child Protection Committee (ACPC). The ACPC has a statutory role in child protection. This includes:

- development of local Child Protection guidelines;
- auditing the performance of child protection procedures;
- promotion of the development of good interagency cooperation and training;
- investigation of cases where child protection has failed.

The ACPC should, as a minimum, contain members from social services, education, health, the police, probation services and the National Society for the Prevention of Cruelty to Children (NSPCC). The report goes on to document the detailed organization of the ACPC.

The report continues by detailing the way in which child protection procedures are intended to operate. Referrals should be made to the Social Services department, which has a duty to investigate. Social Services in turn may involve the police if they believe a criminal act has occurred, though Social Services may, if it is felt to be in the best interests of the child, continue to lead the investigation. Should the child be felt to be at risk of 'significant harm', then Social Services must invoke the statutory child protection powers following a strategy discussion between Social Services, the police and other involved agencies. One power not in the Children Act, but in the Family Law Act 1996 is an exclusion order. This order allows the exclusion of a perpetrator from the home, rather than having to remove the child, allowing the child to remain with its family.

Following further enquiries, and always within 15 working days, an initial child protection conference is held. This conference is intended to decide if the child is at continuing risk of significant harm, and if so, whether the protection of the child requires a formal child protection plan.

The child protection register and its operation is described. Children on the register are considered to be at continuing risk of significant harm. Decisions about continuing risk of significant harm are made at a review child protection conference. Children are to be removed from the register when they reach 18 years of age or permanently move out of the local authority area.

The document describes the underlying principles of child protection and concludes with a description of the intended operation of case reviews and organization of inter-agency training.

REFERENCE

1. *Working Together to Safeguard Children*. Department of Health. The Stationary Office. 1999.

Covert Video Recordings of Life-threatening Child Abuse: Lessons for Child Protection

KEY POINTS

- Described covert video surveillance of 39 children with apparent life-threatening episodes
- Revealed abuse in 33 of the 39 cases
- Described characteristic findings in attempted suffocation
- In the 41 siblings of the patients there had been 12 deaths of which nine were found to be due to abuse
- The majority of the abusing parents had personality disorders
- In all children presenting with apparent life-threatening episodes, child abuse should be considered
- Attempted strangulation often results in facial petechiae

This controversial paper was produced in late 1997 [1] and became a focus of attention for the news media. It described, in graphic detail, the observations made at two UK hospitals, while covertly observing 39 children. Thirty-six had a history of apparent life-threatening episodes (ALTEs), one had fabricated epilepsy, one had severe failure to thrive, and in one case strangulation was suspected. The observations took place over a period of 10 years. The methods are described in detail within the paper. They essentially involved the use of four cameras observing the child from all angles, and the use of observers at all times. The children were continuously monitored with pulse oximetry, electrocardiography (ECG) and respiratory movement monitors. Key points concerning the observations were:

- the parents were unaware of the audio-visual monitoring;
- observation was done with the cooperation of the police;
- the children were observed, rather than the parents;
- help was rapidly available if abuse was observed.

The results section describes each of the surveillance findings in detail. Many of the observations were disturbing. Thirty parents were observed intentionally suffocating their child. Key findings in intentional suffocation were described as:

- petechial haemorrhages – facial, conjunctival and on the throat;
- bleeding from the nose or mouth;
- an increased lymphocyte count was observed after some events.

The observed abuse was premeditated and without provocation. The classically described picture of the fretful child 'winding up' the parents was not observed. These were not isolated events.

The authors suggest that in all cases of ALTE, there should be a high index of suspicion of child abuse.

Psychiatric assessments of many of the abusing parents showed them to have personality disorders. Given the current views on the untreatability of these problems this has implications for the management of child abuse in the community.

There have been several subsequent letters and articles, in various journals, which have criticized the ethical basis of covert video surveillance.

REFERENCE

1. Southall DP, Banks MW, Samuels MP. Covert video recordings of life-threatening child abuse: lessons for child protection. *Pediatrics* 1997; **100**: 735–760.

INTERNATIONAL POLICY

The State of the World's Children

KEY POINTS

- Annual report produced by UNICEF
- Different topics of importance to the welfare of children are considered each year
- Detailed economic and social statistics are given for each country in the world
- The 1999 report focused on education
- Reports on which children are receiving education and which are not
- Makes recommendations to improve education, especially for girls and minority groups

UNICEF produces this annual report which looks at issues which affect the welfare of the world's children. It can be divided into two main parts. In the first part, a different topic (or topics) of importance to children's welfare is considered each year. For example, in the 1996 report the question of children in war was examined. The report included a statement of UNICEF's anti-war agenda. There was also a more detailed discussion of issues raised and accounts from children of their own experiences. The 2000 report is set to look at a child's rights.

In 1999, 'The State of The World's Children' focused on education, reporting on the efforts of the international community to create an 'education revolution' with the aim of education for all [1].

In 1959, the General Assembly of the UN adopted the Declaration on the Rights of the Child, declaring education as a basic right of all people. Education is the single most powerful way of 'combating poverty, empowering women, safeguarding children from exploitative and hazardous labour and sexual exploitation, and controlling population growth'. Since 1959, education rates have improved, primary enrolment rates doubling or tripling in many countries, but there are currently 130 million children (21%) in the developing world who do not have access to basic education of whom two-thirds are girls; almost one-sixth of the world's population is illiterate, the majority being women.

The first chapter is divided into three sections: the right to education, the education revolution, and investing in human rights. In each section there are many illustrations of the issues by reference to schemes in individual countries.

THE RIGHT TO EDUCATION

Article 28 of the 1989 UN Convention on The Rights of a Child [2] (see also pages 48–49) states that all children have the right to an education – primary education should be compulsory and available to all, secondary education should be available and accessible to all children. Article 29 states that 'a child's education should be directed to the development of the child's personality, talents, and mental and physical abilities to their fullest potential'. Article 12 states that children have the right to freedom of expression in matters which affect them. This was a widely ratified convention and is now a binding international law. As detailed above, these rights are not being enforced throughout the developing world.

There is a strong correlation between education and mortality rates, particularly child mortality. A 10% increase in girls going to primary school correlates to a reduction in infant mortality rate of 4.1 deaths per 1000, and in going to secondary school by a further 5.6 deaths per 1000. Schooling also results in significant reductions in birth rates.

Tens of millions of children are denied education because they work full time, often in hazardous and exploitative conditions. Others have no school to attend, or schools with too few teachers, or poor teachers, or schools lacking in books and supplies. It is noted that the quality of education provided is as important as simply providing it. Poor education results in high dropout rates. Unfortunately, resources are scarce in the developing world and in many places there are not even the most basic facilities such as chalkboards or light other than daylight. Overcrowding is common and in the worst places there may be 60–90 children in one class. Within these confines, teaching is difficult and some teachers resort to corporal punishment and rigid discipline. The subject matter is often irrelevant to the children's daily lives and future needs. In some countries, such as those in Eastern Europe, the enrolment rate is actually falling, a result of poor organization of the education systems there.

The Convention on the Rights of the Child also makes it clear that there should be no discrimination. To this end, schools in the developing world need to work particularly on promoting education for girls. Armed conflicts cause difficulties in education, not least because they soak up vast amounts of money, and educational per capita expenditure has halved over the last 20 years. However, many countries are trying hard to improve their education systems and some are basing reforms on the Convention on the Rights of a Child. These changes mark the beginnings of an educational revolution.

THE EDUCATION REVOLUTION

Over the last 10 years, consensus has grown about changes needed to improve learning and these changes are being put into practice internationally. This is being described as 'the education revolution' which has five key elements.

1. **Learning for life:** approaches to teaching designed to make education more fulfilling and relevant, with the instillation of a life-long love of learning. Teachers are seen as facilitators rather than 'dictators of fact'. Children should leave school equipped with basic literacy, numeracy and life skills – e.g. cooperation, communication. They should be encouraged to think for themselves. There should be opportunities for joy and play. Health is an important aspect, with children in developing countries fighting frequent respiratory, gastrointestinal and other illnesses resulting in lost schooling and possible permanent impairment of learning. This may be lessened by health promotion campaigns such as those instigated in Egypt, e.g. school medicals, nutrition programmes, free health insurance for school children.

2. **Access, quality and flexibility:** aiming to reach the children 'on the margins of the education system – girls, disabled, ethnic minorities and child labourers' by making schools more accessible and education more flexible. Children in many remote areas access education by distance learning involving the radio, television and audiotapes. It is recommended that children be taught in their mother tongue as this speeds up the learning process. The majority of children not being schooled are working, often doing domestic or agricultural labour. Most of these children want to go to school, but the economic impact on their families is too great. In some parts of the world, e.g. Brazil, educational grants are being offered to the lowest income families to help combat this.
3. **Schools should be safe,** stimulating environments with safe water and decent sanitation. Teachers should be motivated and the curricula should be relevant.
4. **Gender sensitivity and girls' education:** the education of girls is a top priority which needs to be addressed at cultural and political levels. Educating girls has a profound socio-economic impact – reduced infant and child mortality, better child nutrition, less childhood illness, lower birth rate, lower intrapartum death rate and greater life choices including the ability to play a role in a country's politics and economics. Gender bias in teaching should be eliminated and classrooms should be child-friendly places where girls and boys can contribute equally.
5. **The state as a key partner:** education for all requires the commitment of governments to meet the educational rights as stated in the Convention on the Rights of a Child. Governments need to coordinate all the elements of their education system to create cohesive and flexible education for all. This should include more opportunities for girls, ethnic minorities and disabled children. Governments need to work in partnership with local communities and parents. In many countries more money is spent per capita on higher education than on primary education. This imbalance needs to be rectified.

CARE FOR THE YOUNG CHILD

In 1990, the World Conference on Education for All presented a global consensus on an expanded vision of basic education. It made the point that learning begins at birth and described evidence which suggests that the quality of care during the first few years of a child's life can have a long-lasting effect on brain development. Research shows that the most effective way to nurture and stimulate is by providing good, structured day care outside the home, benefiting both the child and the national economy.

In the second part of the report, statistics relating to economic and social issues are presented for each country. They cover a large number of areas including:

- basic national statistics, e.g. total population, life expectancy, infant mortality;
- nutritional statistics, e.g. percentage of breast feeding mothers;
- health statistics, e.g. percentage of fully immunized children;
- educational statistics, e.g. primary and secondary school enrolment;
- demographic statistics, e.g. percentage of population living in urban areas;

- economic statistics, e.g. gross national product;
- women related statistics, e.g. attendance of trained personnel at births;
- basic indicators of less populous countries;
- regional summaries.

REFERENCES

1. *The State of the World's Children*. UNICEF, United Nations. 1989.
2. *The UN Convention on the Rights of the Child, 1989*. UK Committee for UNICEF. 1995.

UN Convention on the Rights of a Child

KEY POINTS
- Forms the basis of international law as it relates to children
- Ratified by the UK Government in 1991
- Contains 54 articles, which state the rights of every person up to the age of 18 or majority
- Rights divided into four categories: survival, development, protection and participation

This Convention was adopted by the United Nations General assembly on November 20, 1989, and came into force as international law in 1990 [1]. It follows on from the 1959 UN Declaration on the Rights of a Child, which had no force of law. It contains 54 articles providing a set of principles and standards, which must be taken into account when dealing with children and young people up to the age of 18 years or the age of majority. The Convention was ratified by the British Government in 1991.

The articles can be summarized into four broad categories.

- Survival rights: from the right to life to the provision of basic needs such as food, shelter and health care.
- Development rights: things that children need to reach their full potential such as education, play, conscience and religion.
- Protection rights: the safeguarding of children from all forms of abuse, neglect and exploitation.
- Participation rights: such as the right to free expression.

A number of the articles are of particular relevance to the practice of paediatrics.

Article 3 states that 'in actions concerning children the best interests of the child shall be a primary consideration', a principle embodied in the UK in the 1989 Children Act [2] (see also pages 4–5).

Article 23 covers the rights of disabled children stating the need to recognize their special needs and to extend assistance to them to enable them to enjoy 'a full and decent life'.

Article 24 covers health and health services. It states that all children have the right to 'the enjoyment of the highest attainable standard of health' (subject to the maximum extent of available resources, outlined in article 4). It places particular emphasis on the requirement to provide primary health care, access for parents and children to health education, and to the development of preventative health care.

The UNICEF publication contains the full text of the Convention. This is followed by an easy to understand interpretation of these rights, written by a 9-year-old child for children to read. In addition, there is the text of the UK Declarations and Reservations in their adoption of the Convention. These relate primarily to immigration and young offenders.

REFERENCES

1. *The UN Convention on the Rights of the Child, 1989.* UK Committee for UNICEF. 1995.
2. *The Children Act 1989.* The Stationary Office. 1989.

CLINICAL PRACTICE AND GUIDELINES

Standards for the Development of Clinical Guidelines in Paediatrics and Child Health

KEY POINTS

- Recommendations made to ensure good quality clinical guidelines
- Endorsement criteria required by Quality of Practice Committee (QPC) of the RCPCH
- QPC function described
- College approved guidelines may be publicized in conjunction with NICE

This is the report of the Quality of Practice Committee (QPC) of the Royal College of Paediatrics and Child Health (RCPCH). It was published in 1998 [1].

Over the past decade there has been increasing emphasis on quality and a greater uniformity in the treatment which patients receive. The result of this has been the creation of more clinical guidelines, often in conjunction with audit. The aim of this document is to give guidance on the content, format and development of clinical guidelines. In this way, there will be maximum benefit to paediatricians, purchasers, providers, patients and their carers.

The QPC of the RCPCH is often approached to endorse guidelines developed by certain groups, but can only do this if their explicit guidelines are followed.

The RCPCH has criteria for prioritizing guidelines development. These are divided into primary and secondary criteria. The primary criteria are the degree of public importance, relevance to paediatric practice, availability of evidence-based clinical information and supporting data and susceptibility to health intervention. The secondary criteria include the availability of existing audits which would be useful in developing a guideline, an area in which increased paediatric involvement would be helpful for the field, the high cost of a health intervention, a DoH priority and an area where there is known to be wide variation in clinical practice.

The report uses the Effective Healthcare Bulletin's recommendations that guidelines should be:

- valid so that following guidelines leads to improvements in health;
- reproducible – given the same evidence, other groups would produce similar recommendations;
- reliable – given the same clinical situation, other health professionals would apply them in the same way;
- representative of key disciplines and interests;
- clinically applicable with a defined target population;
- clinically flexible with identified exceptions and ways of incorporating patients' preferences;

- clearly expressed using precise definitions, unambiguous language and user-friendly formats;
- well documented so that participants, assumptions and methods are recorded and recommendations are clearly linked to available evidence;
- scheduled for review – the guidelines should state when and how they will be reviewed.

Development of guidelines often requires a multiprofessional effort. Since it is a complicated process, the report recommends that guideline methodologists should be recruited from the beginning. Comprehensive reviews of the knowledge base are required; this may be something that supervised juniors could do. It provides an evidence-based format. Exactly what the guidelines will cover should be decided in advance. This limits the systematic reviews necessary. The report comments that some guidelines are developed without formal literature reviews, using the expert knowledge and experience of the panel. Once finished, there should be experienced, trained reviewers of the document.

The guidelines should comprise of three essential parts: the guideline report, a quick reference guide and patient information (where appropriate). The guideline report should include how the guidelines were developed, a literature review, an appraisal review document, a review date and a strategy for disseminating its contents.

In addition to prioritizing topics for guideline development, the QPC will give advice and assistance to people wishing to develop guidelines or consensus statements, identify people with enough expertise to appraise the process, make recommendations for endorsement by the RCPCH, formulate strategies for disseminating information and keep a record of the guidelines submitted to or developed by the RCPCH.

When the RCPCH endorses guidelines after formally assessing them, its role should be acknowledged in the document. College approved guidelines will be publicized in the College newsletter, on its guideline database and via the NICE. Some guidelines may be published as College documents.

At the end of the guide is the appraisal form used by the RCPCH to assess guidelines, followed by a user guide for it. This enables potential 'applicants' to ensure they have fulfilled all the necessary criteria for RCPCH endorsement.

REFERENCES

1. Report of the Quality of Practice Committee. *Standards for Development of Clinical Guidelines in Paediatrics and Child Health: role of the Royal College of Paediatrics and Child Health*. London: Royal College of Paediatrics and Child Health. 1998.

FURTHER READING

1. *Implementing clinical practice guidelines: Can guidelines be used to improve clinical practice?* Effective Health Care. 1994.
2. *A First Class Service: Quality in the New NHS*. Department of Health. 1998. (see also pages 12–14).

Medicines For Children

KEY POINTS

- There has been no fully comprehensive and widely accepted formulary available previously
- Many drugs used for children are used off licence or without a product licence
- Not purely a formulary – guidance on how and when to treat with many suggested treatment regimens
- System-based section for advice on specific disease processes
- Includes neonatal information

This book was published in 1999 by the RCPCH [1].

Many of the drugs used for children are used outside the conditions in the product licence as there is often no suitable alternative. Product licences only control marketing and not prescription of drugs. This has lead to much uncertainty and confusion when prescribing and administering drugs to children. Over the years, formularies have been produced by various hospitals and institutions which are helpful, but have differing advice and drug dosages. This comprehensive guide to the use of drugs in children has been produced through consensus opinion to 'meet the need for accessible, sound information and guidance'.

The introductory chapter lists some of the Acts and statements relevant to prescribing for children. The conclusions of the Standing Committee on Medicines (a joint committee of the RCPCH and the Neonatal and Paediatric Pharmacists Group) are listed below.

- Those who prescribe for a child should choose the medicine which offers the best prospect for that child with due regard for cost.
- The informed use of licensed medicines for unlicensed applications or unlicensed medicines is necessary for paediatric practice.
- In general it is not necessary to obtain the explicit consent of parents, carers or child patients to prescribe or administer licensed medicines for unlicensed applications or unlicensed medicines.
- NHS trusts and health authorities should support therapeutic practices that are advocated by a respectable, responsible body of professional opinion.

The formulary is divided into several sections which are system based, followed by the formulary itself which lists drugs alphabetically by their generic names. The following is a brief summary of some of the contents.

Giving medicines

Gives advice on which route and in which form medicines should be given and why, including helpful advice on the practicalities of actually getting a child to take medicine.

Life support
Brief guidance on treatment of asystole and anaphylaxis. The guidelines for other emergency treatments are in other relevant sections, e.g. status epilepticus is in the section on neurology.

Poisoning
A list of the phone numbers of the National Poisons Information Service. Guidance on how to assess lethality and the principles of treating poisoning. There is also a description of a number of more common poisonings and their specific treatments, e.g. carbon monoxide poisoning.

Pain management
Guidance on medical and non-drug management of pain, such as providing children with adequate information and performing painful procedures in as friendly an environment as possible. There is also a section on the management of opioid side effects such as pruritis, respiratory depression and nausea. Advice is given on the management of neuropathic pain and the pain due to muscle spasms. The use of anaesthetic agents, sedation and pre-medication is also discussed.

Infections
This is a lengthy section which gives advice regarding length of treatment, route of administration and prophylaxis. It details specific diseases, likely organisms and suggested antibiotic regimens, including neonatal infections. There are separate tables for children with HIV infection and for those who are immunosuppressed.

Nutrition
Nutritional requirements of children of different ages and the feeds available to fulfil these needs or to supplement the diet. There is also a section on parenteral feeding with a run-down on the different preparations available.

Intravenous fluid therapy
Maintenance and replacement fluid regimens are discussed with advice on which fluid to use and how. There is also a section on the use of colloids which advises the use of normal saline for rapid volume expansion in resuscitation and discusses the use of synthetic gelatines in neonates and children.

System-based sections
These sections look at some important or difficult areas of medical treatment such as the step-up, step-down management of asthma (in line with the British Thoracic Society Guidelines; see also pages 58–61), the emergency treatment of cardiac dysrhythmias, recurrent abdominal pain, nocturnal enuresis, nephrotic syndrome, the use of growth hormone and the treatment of sleep disorders.

Formulary
Drugs are listed in alphabetical order with indications, dosages for different ages and details of contra-indications and side effects. Some drug listings, such as that for paracetamol, also include advice on the treatment of overdose.

REFERENCE

1. Hull D, ed. *Medicines for Children*. London: Royal College of Paediatrics and Child Health. 1999.

Immunization Against Infectious Disease

KEY POINTS

- Invaluable source of practical information
- Covers general issues relating to immunization and details of specific vaccines
- Gives the recommended immunization schedule

This guide to immunization against infectious diseases was first published in 1992 by the HMSO on behalf of the Department of Health, the Welsh Office, the Scottish Office Department of Health and the DHSS (Northern Ireland) [1]. The current edition was published in 1996. It is widely known as 'the green book'.

The guide is intended as a valuable resource of information for all health care professionals involved in immunization in the UK: doctors, health visitors, etc. The Chief Medical Officer sends recently updated information, such as that on meningococcal immunization, to all doctors. Although there is some information on travel vaccines, detailed risks and recommendations for each country are provided in the companion book 'Health Information for Overseas Travel' [2].

The guide can be divided into two main parts. In the first part, general issues relating to immunization are considered. These include:

- The basic principles of immunity: for example, inducing primary and secondary vaccination responses by a series of injections, the use of adjuvants such as aluminium phosphate to enhance the antibody response and the differences between active and passive immunity.
- Consent: emphasizing that it must always be obtained, in writing or verbally. In line with consent for other reasons, children who understand the implications of the vaccination, but who are under 16-years-old, may provide or refuse consent for themselves.
- Storage of vaccines: recommending a designated person be responsible, and that vaccines should not be stored in domestic fridges or with food/drink.
- Immunization procedures: this advice is based on the recommendations of the Joint Committee of Vaccination and Immunization (JCVI). It details how to check that the vaccine to be used is appropriate, how to reconstitute vaccines with diluents and how to actually inject the vaccine, be it intradermal, subcutaneous or intramuscular. There is a picture showing where the vaccine should be injected and which needle sizes to use. The section on administration of intradermal Bacillus de Calmette-Guérin (BCG) vaccine is particularly detailed with advice to expect significant resistance and the formation of a 7-mm bleb when correctly given. Nurses may give immunizations when trained in immunization and treatment of anaphylaxis.
- Indications and contraindications: some groups, e.g. premature babies or those with HIV, are at increased risk of complication from infectious disease and should be immunized as a priority. Children coming into the UK with an unknown vaccination status should be assumed not to be immunized and should therefore receive a full course of immunizations. Some people with medical conditions, e.g.

hyposplenism, are at increased risk of certain infections and the guide details who should receive which vaccines. The guide also lists groups who should not receive certain vaccines, e.g. patients undergoing chemotherapy should not have live vaccines. Other general contraindications to immunization such as previous severe reaction are listed. A history of allergy is not a contra-indication, though anaphylaxis to egg is a contraindication to flu and yellow fever vaccination. There is increasing evidence that the measles, mumps and rubella (MMR) vaccine can be given safely to children even if there is a history of anaphylaxis to eggs. There is a specific section on immunization of people with HIV infection.

- Adverse reactions including anaphylaxis: these should be reported in the usual way using the yellow cards. Where possible, the batch number should be given. Most suspected reactions are minor, e.g. rash, fever. In 1995 there were 152 reports classified as serious reactions – compared with over 14 million vaccinations given that year. This equates to a serious reaction in every 100 000 doses of vaccine given. Some vaccines are associated with particular adverse reactions, for example, MMR may cause thrombocytopaenia. Recommendations for treatment of anaphylaxis are given, but it should be noted that these have changed since publication (see also pages 74, 75).
- Vaccine damage payments scheme: this provides a one off lump sum for people suffering a physical or mental disablement of 80% or more resulting from vaccination of themselves or of their mother whilst pregnant, with diphtheria, tetanus, polio, pertussis, measles, rubella, tuberculosis, mumps or HIB. It is not compensation, but it is designed to make life easier.
- The recommended UK immunization schedule in 1996.
- Immunization of laboratory staff: detailing which vaccinations are recommended and for whom.

Of note, the Council of the Faculty of Homeopathy strongly supports the immunization programme and recommends that immunization should be given unless medically contraindicated.

The second part looks at specific vaccines. The information about each vaccine includes:

- background information (including some epidemiology) on the disease;
- details of the vaccine, e.g. live or toxoid, etc;
- recommendations for its use: who and when to administer it, dose and route of administration;
- adverse reactions and contraindications;
- other issues specific to a vaccine or disease, e.g. prophylaxis for invasive HIB disease/meningococcal infection;
- details of suppliers.

The book concludes with a list of Child Health Department contacts by region. The back page has colour photographs of each grade of reaction following Heaf testing.

REFERENCES

1. *1996 Immunization Against Infectious Disease*. The Stationary Office. 1996.
2. *Health Information for Overseas Travel*. The Stationary Office. 1995.

Asthma in Adults and Schoolchildren

KEY POINTS

- Stepwise approach to the management of asthma
- Aiming for symptom control and then a reduction of medication once control is established
- Patient education, including the use of asthma plans recommended
- Suggests criteria for admission to, and discharge from, hospital

One of two papers issued in 1997 as a review of the 1993 British Thoracic Society Guidelines [1,2]. It covers the management of asthma in adults and children over 5 years of age, and is intended for use by both GPs and paediatricians.

The guidelines emphasize the importance of ensuring the diagnosis of asthma is correct, especially in a patient who does not respond to treatment. These patients should be referred to a specialist.

The stepwise approach recommended in the management of asthma is listed below.

1. Occasional use of inhaled short acting β_2 agonists.
2. Regular low dose inhaled steroid plus inhaled short acting β_2 agonists as required. A trial of chromoglycate (or nedocromil) can be used but, if unsuccessful, inhaled steroids should be introduced.
3. High dose inhaled steroids or low dose inhaled steroid plus inhaled long-acting β_2 agonist. Inhaled short acting β_2 agonists as required.
4. High dose inhaled steroids plus one of
   - long acting β_2 agonists;
   - slow release theophylline;
   - inhaled ipratropium;
   - high dose inhaled bronchodilators;
   - chromoglycate or nedocromil.
5. Addition of regular steroid tablets.

It may be necessary to start at a high step and then 'step-down' once symptoms are controlled.

In this context, low dose inhaled steroid is beclomethasone or budesonide 100–400 µg twice daily or fluticasone 50–200 µg twice daily. High dose inhaled steroid corresponds to beclomethasone or budesonide 400–1000 µg twice daily or fluticasone 200–500 µg twice daily.

The role of each of the therapeutic agents is discussed in greater detail. The use of new chlorofluorocarbon (CFC)-free propellants is discussed, and it is recommended that patients be reassured that old inhalers were changed because they were damaging to the environment, not the patients. The exacerbating effect on asthma of passive smoking is discussed.

Clear written asthma plans are required. They should indicate the action required when symptoms worsen. The management of young children should be based on symptoms rather than peak flows.

The management of acute severe asthma and life-threatening features are highlighted (cyanosis, peak expiratory flow (PEF) <33% of best or predicted, silent chest, exhaustion, agitation or reduced level of consciousness).

Prior to discharge from hospital, patients should have been on their discharge medicine for 24 h, with a PEF >75% of predicted or best and a diurnal variation of <25%. Oral steroid courses should be completed following discharge from hospital and GP follow-up should be within 1 week.

REFERENCES

1. British Thoracic Society, National Asthma Campaign, *et al*. Asthma in adults and schoolchildren. *Thorax* 1997; **52**: S2–8.
2. British Thoracic Society, British Paediatric Association, Royal College of Physicians of London, The King's Fund Centre, National Asthma Campaign, *et al*. Asthma in children under 5 years of age. *Thorax* 1993; **48**: S1–24.

Asthma in Children Under 5 Years of Age

KEY POINTS
- Management of children under 5 years differs from older children and adults
- Suggests a stepwise approach to the management of chronic asthma
- Based upon few clinical trials
- Gives management guidelines for acute severe exacerbations

The second of two papers issued as a review of the 1993 British Thoracic Society Guidelines. This paper covers the management of asthma in children under 5 years of age [1] (see also pages 58–59).

The paper starts by discussing the nature of asthma in these children and how repeated episodes of viral-induced wheeze represent a distinct clinical entity from atopic asthma.

The role of drugs in the management of asthma is explored, and in particular the risk/benefit analysis for the use of inhaled steroids, overall being in favour of their use. A table of appropriate starting doses is provided.

A useful table of age appropriate inhaler devices is provided. Broadly the use of a metered dose inhaler (MDI) with spacer device is best up to the age of 5 years, with a face mask added for those under 2 years.

The steps recommended in the management of asthma in children under 5 years are:
- occasional use of inhaled short-acting β_2 agonists;
- regular inhaled preventer, either chromoglycate or low dose inhaled steroid;
- higher dose inhaled steroids. Consider adding long acting β_2 agonists or slow release oral theophylline;
- high dose inhaled steroids and regular bronchodilators. The bronchodilators may be long acting β_2 agonists, slow release xanthines, or nebulized β_2 agonists.

Chromoglycate can be administered as powder (20 mg, 3–4 times daily) or via an MDI (10 mg, three times daily). Low dose inhaled steroids can be beclomethasone or budesonide up to 400 μg daily or fluticasone up to 200 μg daily. High dose inhaled steroids can be beclomethasone or budesonide up to 800 μg daily or fluticasone up to 500 μg daily. A 5-day course of oral prednisolone can be used to gain control.

The management of acute severe asthma is discussed. There is more emphasis on clinical judgement than objective measurements in contrast with adults. Severe features are:
- too breathless to feed or talk;
- respiratory rate >50 breaths min⁻¹;
- pulse >140 beats min⁻¹;

- use of accessory muscles;
- arterial oxygen saturation (SaO$_2$) <92% in air.

These children need immediate intervention and admission to hospital. High flow oxygen should be used. Nebulized salbutamol (2.5–5 mg) driven by oxygen should be given, and oral prednisolone administered (1–2 mg kg^{-1} day^{-1}, 20 mg day^{-1} over 1 year of age).

Life-threatening features are:

- cyanosis;
- silent chest;
- fatigue, exhaustion or poor respiratory effort;
- agitation or reduced level of consciousness.

Poor response to bronchodilators, or the presence of life-threatening features should result in the starting of intravenous aminophylline (with loading dose if not using oral theophylline). Nebulized ipratropium should also be added.

Patients who deteriorate with progression of life-threatening features should be transferred to an intensive care unit accompanied by a doctor prepared to intubate.

Patients who are recovering from an episode of acute severe asthma should have been stable on their discharge medication for 6–8 hours. Oral steroid courses should be completed at home. Parents should be given a clear written asthma plan. Open access to the ward should be available for the 24 h following discharge should the child deteriorate.

REFERENCE

1. British Thoracic Society, British Paediatric Association, Royal College of Physicians of London, The King's Fund Centre, National Asthma Campaign, *et al*. Asthma in children under 5 years of age. *Thorax* 1993; **48**: S1–24.

The Effect of Intensive Treatment of Diabetes on the Development and Progression of Long Term Complications in Insulin-Dependent Diabetes Mellitus

KEY POINTS

- Large multicentre randomized clinical trial
- Compared intensive therapy with conventional therapy
- Intensive therapy reduces the incidence and progression of complications of IDDM (retinopathy, nephropathy, and neuropathy)
- Intensive therapy also results in greater weight gain and increased frequency of hypoglycaemic episodes

Published in 1993, this paper reports on the findings of the Diabetes Control and Complications Trial (DCCT) [1]. It confirmed what clinicians had always believed but had no concrete evidence for, that the long-term complications of insulin-dependent diabetes mellitus (IDDM) could be reduced or delayed through improved diabetic control.

The DCCT was a multicentre, randomized clinical trial carried out between 1983 and 1989. It recruited 1441 patients between the ages of 13 and 39 years with IDDM who had no severe diabetic complications. The patients were divided into two cohorts on the basis of their retinal status, either no retinopathy (the primary prevention cohort) or mild to moderate non-proliferative retinopathy (the secondary intervention cohort). Treatment was randomized to conventional therapy or intensive therapy. Conventional therapy involved the use of once or twice daily insulin, with daily monitoring of blood or urinary glucose and follow-up every 3 months.

Intensive therapy involved three or more daily doses of insulin (or the use of an insulin infusion) combined with four or more daily measurements of blood glucose. Insulin dosages were modified according to the results of blood glucose monitoring and predicted requirements. Monthly follow-up was used, with further telephone advice. The aim of intensive therapy was a preprandial blood glucose between 3.9 and 6.7 mmol l^{-1} and postprandial level of less than 10 mmol l^{-1} and a normal glycosylated haemoglobin (Hb A_{1c}). Despite the intensive intervention, less than 5% of the intensive therapy cohort achieved an average Hb A_{1c} in the normal range.

The long-term complications of IDDM, retinopathy, nephropathy and neuropathy were observed in each of the cohorts.

In the primary prevention cohort, the incidence of retinopathy was reduced by 76% through the use of intensive therapy. The progression of retinopathy in the secondary intervention cohort was also reduced by 54% by the use of intensive therapy.

Nephropathy, defined as the development of microalbuminuria, was reduced by 34% through the use of intensive therapy in the primary prevention cohort and by 43% in the secondary intervention cohort.

The development of neuropathy was similarly reduced through the use of intensive therapy, by 69% in the primary prevention cohort.

These beneficial effects of intensive therapy were balanced by a large increase (greater than 3-fold) in the number of severe hypoglycaemic episodes in the intensive therapy cohort. There was also a 33% increase in the incidence of becoming overweight in the intensive therapy cohort.

The paper concludes by recommending that most patients with IDDM should be treated with intensive therapy regimes, with the aim of achieving blood glucose levels in the normal range.

Children under 13 years of age were not included in this trial. The risks of severe hypoglycaemia for neurodevelopment in this age group need to be balanced against the risk of diabetic complications.

REFERENCE

1. The Diabetes Control and Complications Trial Research Group. The effect of intensive treatment of diabetes on the development and progression of long-term complications in insulin-dependent diabetes mellitus. *N Engl J Med* 1993; **329**: 977–986.

Clinical Opinion – Imaging in Urinary Tract Infection

KEY POINTS

- Makes recommendations about urinary tract imaging following a proven urinary tract infection (UTI)
- No single correct way to investigate
- Renal scarring may be prevented/limited by early diagnosis and treatment of UTI and/or vesicoureteric reflux (VUR)
- Screening of siblings for VUR may prevent scarring

The British Paediatric Association (now RCPCH) Standing Committee on Paediatric Practice Guidelines published this document in 1996 [1]. It replaces the 1991 guidelines.

Urinary tract infections (UTI) are common in children. Over the past 20 years there has been significant controversy about when and in whom to perform urinary tract imaging following proven UTI in children [2]. The result of this has been a wide variation in the type and timing of imaging performed with the possible end result of renal damage remaining unidentified. These guidelines drawn up by a reputable panel aim to consolidate opinion and create a sensible formula to guide physicians dealing with children with proven UTI. The document points out that there is no single correct way to investigate, but gives the rationale behind performing each of the investigations and provides suggested guidelines.

The two main issues surrounding imaging are that renal damage may occur early and is usually caused by untreated infection, usually in the presence of vesicoureteric reflux (VUR), and that renal scarring may be prevented/limited by early diagnosis and treatment. In addition, the identification of VUR in a child may allow the screening of any siblings and thereby prevention of scarring before infection occurs. This may also be possible if investigations are performed postnatally in children with antenatally-detected hydronephrosis.

The paper suggests the following initial investigations with the obvious proviso that further investigation may be necessary depending on the clinical situation and in the presence of recurrent infections.

Children aged 0–1 years:

- ultrasound scan (USS) of urinary tract;
- micturating cystourethrogram (MCUG);
- dimercapto succinic acid (DMSA) scan;
- if there is significant hydronephrosis in the absence of VUR a paediatric nephrology opinion should be sought. The paper makes the comments that some physicians would advocate the use of these investigations in children up to 2 years of age.

Children aged 1–5 years:

- USS of urinary tract;
- DMSA scan (although some physicians would use DMSA selectively as in those over 5 years);
- cystography if DMSA is abnormal, if there is a family history of reflux nephropathy, if there is evidence of upper tract involvement, or if infections are recurrent.

Children aged over 5 years, the clinical opinion document suggests the division of patients into those with cystitis/lower tract symptoms and those with systemic symptoms (as described by Rickwood *et al.* [2]):

- lower tract symptoms: USS of urinary tract and/or abdominal X-ray;
- systemic symptoms: USS of urinary tract and/or abdominal X-ray; DMSA (and cystography if DMSA shows scarring).

The document gives a brief summary of the pros and cons of each investigation and what each one is useful in demonstrating. It also points out the controversy surrounding the timing of DMSA scanning which should not be performed until 6 weeks after infection to prevent detection of abnormalities which will resolve. If there is any evidence of calculi, such as renal colic or Proteus infection, or there is suspicion of neuropathic bladder, then an abdominal X-ray should be performed. Where MCUG is being performed, the urine should be free from infection but there is no necessity for an absolute time delay. Because of the high risk of introducing infection during MCUG, all children with demonstrable reflux should be started on a course of antibiotics.

The document recommends the use of prophylactic antibiotics until investigations are complete in all children under 1 year of age and also in children over 1 year in whom cystography is indicated.

REFERENCES

1. *Clinical Opinion: Imaging in Urinary Tract Infection.* London: British Paediatric Association. 1996.
2. Rickwood A, Carty HM, McKendrick T, *et al.* Current imaging of childhood urinary tract infections: prospective survey. *BMJ* 1992; **304**: 663–665.

Consensus Statement on Management and Audit Potential for Steroid Responsive Nephrotic Syndrome

KEY POINTS

- Gives criteria for diagnosis of steroid sensitive nephrotic syndrome
- Unified step-wise approach to management with steroids
- Identifies patients in whom alternative treatments should be considered
- Indicates when to refer to a regional nephrology centre
- Defines audit points for evaluation of practice

Produced by the British Association of Paediatric Nephrology and the Research Unit of the Royal College of Physicians in 1994, this was a landmark document in that it drew together disparate opinion on the management of steroid sensitive nephrotic syndrome (SSNS) and produced a unified approach to its management [1]. The report was aimed at general paediatricians, who manage the majority of cases of SSNS.

The report defines nephrotic syndrome as oedema, in the presence of a plasma albumin <25 g l^{-1} and proteinuria >40 mg m^{-2} h^{-1} or a protein/creatinine ratio >200 mg $mmol^{-1}$. Definitions of remission, relapse, frequent relapses, steroid dependence and steroid resistance are also given in the report.

A flow chart showing the sequence of management is given, and this provides a stepwise approach to the management of relapses on and off treatment. Steroid doses are recommended and the patients in whom alternative treatments should be considered are identified.

There are 16 audit points given in the report and these outline the recommended management of SSNS, and provide a standard for audit. The key points are listed below.

- Diagnosis should be confirmed by the quantitative analysis of proteinuria.
- Height and blood pressure should be recorded initially and at each outpatient attendance.
- Initial investigations should include urinalysis, culture, early morning protein/creatinine ratio. Blood tests should include plasma electrolytes, creatinine, protein, a full blood count and test for Hepatitis B surface antigen.
- The currently recommended treatment for the initial episode and for the first two relapses is prednisolone 60 mg m^{-2} day^{-1} (to a maximum of 80 mg day^{-1}) until in remission, and then 40 mg m^{-2} day^{-1} (to a maximum of 60 mg per dose) alternate days for 4 weeks, and then stop.
- Patients should be given a steroid warning card.
- Remissions and relapses should be clearly documented, as should decisions about alternative treatments (cyclophosphamide, levamisole and cyclosporin). Clear

explanations should be given to parents and the child about the risks of these treatments.
- A specialist paediatric nephrologists' opinion should be sought in steroid resistant, steroid dependent and frequently relapsing cases, before the use of alternative treatments.
- Renal biopsy should only be performed in an appropriate regional centre.

Other management points made in the report include dietary advice, the use of prophylactic penicillin whilst oedematous, and the treatment of hypovolaemia.

The complications of nephrotic syndrome and its treatment are discussed at length. In particular the prevention of varicella zoster virus is discussed and the indications for varicella zoster immunoglobulin (VZIG) and aciclovir are given. Advice is also given regarding immunizations.

REFERENCE

1. Report of a workshop by the British Association for Paediatric Nephrology and Research Unit, Royal College of Physicians. Consensus statement on management and audit potential for steroid responsive nephrotic syndrome. *Arch Dis Child* 1994; **70**: 151–157.

Reducing Mother-to-Child Transmission of HIV Infection in the UK

KEY POINTS

- Two-thirds of all HIV infections in children could be prevented by maternal anti-retroviral treatment in combination with abstaining from breast feeding
- Effective treatment can only be offered if HIV infection is diagnosed before or during pregnancy
- Over 75% of HIV infection in pregnant women is undiagnosed by the time of birth
- Most pregnant women who know that they are HIV-positive opt for interventions to reduce transmission
- Report recommends that women in high prevalence areas and those at high risk should be offered routine antenatal HIV testing
- Professionals need to be educated about HIV in pregnancy and its implications for mother and child

This document contains the recommendations of an intercollegiate working party for enhancing voluntary HIV testing in pregnancy. It was published in 1998 by the RCPCH [1].

In light of the fact that treating mothers infected with HIV reduces HIV transmission to their babies, this working party was set up in 1997 to look at ways of reducing maternally acquired HIV infection in children. Amongst others, the working party included representatives from the Royal Colleges (Paediatrics and Child Health, obstetrics and gynaecology, GPs, physicians, nursing and midwifery), as well as representatives of ethnic minorities and HIV-positive women.

Anonymous testing of pregnant women has shown that there are about 300 babies born to HIV-positive women each year in the UK. In only 12% of cases is the HIV infection known prior to delivery. Over 50% of women discover they are HIV-positive when their child becomes ill and has the diagnosis made. HIV prevalence is highest in London (one in 520 births) with some districts having a prevalence up to one in 170 births. Edinburgh and Dundee also have high prevalence rates, but they also have much higher rates of prenatal diagnosis. Outside London, maternal HIV infection is less common, with an average prevalence of one in 5700 births.

Vertical transmission accounts for 85% of paediatric AIDS patients in the UK. It may occur before, during or after birth. Breast feeding doubles the transmission rate [2] (see also pages 72–73). In the absence of breastfeeding, about two-thirds of infections are acquired around the time of delivery. Giving infected mothers zidovudine antenatally reduces transmission rates from 15–20% to about 5%. Zidovudine is well tolerated in pregnancy and by babies. Its use has significantly reduced the numbers of HIV-positive children in the USA and France; compared to the UK where numbers are still rising.

Routine antenatal HIV testing is being implemented in some European countries and is felt to be especially cost-effective where prevalence is high. In France and the Netherlands, all women are offered antenatal HIV testing. Some developing countries, e.g. Thailand and South Africa are offering antenatal testing in some places.

Zidovudine can be used during pregnancy, labour and in early infancy, and the optimum time to start treatment is not yet clear. It is also unclear whether using zidovudine in pregnancy reduces its efficacy (by inducing viral resistance) when used to treat the mother later on in her illness. Long term consequences for the child treated antenatally/neonatally with zidovudine are not known.

Antenatal detection of HIV is also of benefit to mothers as it will allow them to benefit from treatment with combination therapies.

Currently available HIV testing is highly sensitive and specific. Routine testing in high prevalence areas has been recommended by the DoH since 1992. However, it is still not offered routinely in most London hospitals, and where it is offered, uptake does not correlate with prevalence.

It is felt that HIV infection is different from other antenatal testing as a positive result can have implications which confer disadvantages to the individual, such as rejection by a partner, or health insurance problems. In addition there seems to be a feeling that women would prefer not to know their infection status. This assumption has become indefensible since the advent of effective treatment both to reduce HIV vertical transmission and to treat the mother. When given adequate information about the potential benefits of antenatal HIV testing, most women understand the need for it. Verbal consent is required. Women who test positive urgently require counselling, information and support. Those who test positive usually opt for interventions aimed at reducing transmission. Women should be advised of the need for follow-up of their infants until it is known whether or not they are infected and the fact that the long term effects of zidovudine are not known. Having given a woman all the necessary information, her decision about what treatment, if any, she wishes to have, is final.

The report recommends that all women should be informed about HIV in pregnancy, including ways of reducing transmission. It recommends that those in areas of high prevalence (more than one in 2000 births) or those at higher risk (e.g. those who have injected drugs or whose partners are bisexual) should routinely be offered antenatal HIV testing. It is not clear whether testing should be routinely performed in low prevalence areas and a cost–benefit analysis of this is currently being done. HIV testing should be voluntary, confidential and available alongside other antenatal tests.

The report also recommends that all staff involved in the care of pregnant women should receive education about HIV infection in pregnancy and about possible interventions. The information these professionals receive should be updated regularly.

The report recommends that monitoring of HIV infection in pregnancy should continue, by confidential reporting of positive tests to the Royal College of

Obstetricians and Gynaecologists, to the British Paediatric Surveillance Unit and by the reporting of positive tests from the Public Health Laboratory Service (PHLS).

The working party will reconvene in 2000 to look at these issues again.

REFERENCES

1. *Reducing Mother to Child Transmission of HIV Infection in the UK.* Recommendations of an intercollegiate working party for enhancing voluntary confidential HIV testing in pregnancy. London: Royal College of Paediatrics and Child Health. 1998.
2. *HIV and Infant Feeding – Guidance from the UK Chief Medical Officers' Expert Advisory Group on AIDS.* Department of Health. September 1999.

HIV and Infant Feeding

KEY POINTS

- Most UK HIV-infected children are infected following vertical transmission before or during birth or from breast-feeding
- Refraining from breast-feeding reduces the risk of HIV transmission to the baby from 15–25% to under 5%
- Women should be given access to HIV testing during pregnancy
- HIV-positive women should be given help and advice as early as possible
- Where there is no safe breast milk substitute available it is better to breast-feed; this is unusual in the UK

Published in September 1999 by the DoH, this booklet provides guidance from the UK Chief Medical Officers' Expert Advisory Group on AIDS [1]. Its aim is to help health care professionals give information and advice about infant feeding to women infected with HIV. It was produced in response to evidence that there is a significant risk of vertical transmission of HIV from breast-feeding.

The booklet points out that women will only be able to make informed decisions about ways of protecting their babies if they know their own HIV status. It is therefore important that all pregnant women are offered HIV testing during pregnancy and given adequate information about HIV and its implications for their babies. This should be performed at the earliest opportunity by a health care professional with expertise in this field. Ideally, there should be a key worker to ensure continuity and consistency of advice. The best interests of the baby should be central to any discussions.

The majority of children infected with HIV in the UK are infected following transmission from their mothers. Transmission can be significantly reduced by the use of anti-retroviral treatment, elective Caesarean section and avoiding breast-feeding [2–4] (see also pages 68–70). When breast-feeding is avoided, the risk of HIV transmission from mother to baby falls from 15–25% to under 5%. Transmission rates are higher where mothers are newly infected, probably because of higher viral load. Therefore, mothers who are not infected but who are at risk of becoming infected should be given advice to reduce their risk whilst they are breast-feeding.

In 1997, the WHO issued a statement regarding HIV and infant feeding which stated that all HIV-positive men and women have the right to decide the course of their own reproductive life and to have access to information and services which allow them to protect their family's health. Where children are involved, decisions should be made which are in the best interests of the child. Where there is no possibility of uninterrupted access to suitable and safe breast milk substitutes, it is better to breast-feed despite the risk of HIV transmission. Where a safe, suitable substitute is readily available (as in the UK) this should be used in preference to breast-feeding. The booklet points out that where breast-feeding is the culturally accepted norm it may be difficult for mothers to abstain as this may signal their HIV status. In these situations extra support may be needed.

There may be some mothers who, after considering all the evidence, decide to breast-feed. In these cases she should be given as much information as possible about how to reduce the risk of HIV transmission – early cessation of breast-feeding as soon as a suitable alternative food becomes available, and good positioning at the breast to reduce inflammation such as cracked nipples or mastitis (which may increase the risk of transmission). Where there are breast-feeding problems help should be sought as soon as possible.

REFERENCES

1. *HIV and Infant Feeding – Guidance from the UK Chief Medical Officers' Expert Advisory Group on AIDS*. Department of Health. September 1999.
2. *Reducing Mother to Child Transmission of HIV Infection in the UK*. Recommendations of an intercollegiate working party for enhancing voluntary confidential HIV testing in pregnancy. London: Royal College of Paediatrics and Child Health. 1998.
3. Newell M-L, Gray G, Bryson YJ. Prevention of mother-to-child transmission of HIV-1 infection. *AIDS* 1995; **9**: 107–119.
4. Nicoll A, Newell M-L, Van Praag E, Van de Perre P, Peckham C. *Infant feeding policy and practice in the presence of HIV-1 infection.*

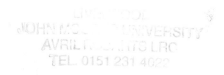

Emergency Medical Treatment of Anaphylactic Reactions

KEY POINTS

- Incidence of anaphylactic reactions is increasing
- It is important to make an accurate diagnosis
- Give oxygen, IM adrenaline, IM/slow IV chlorpheniramine, hydrocortisone and volume expansion if necessary
- Do not use IV adrenaline unless profound, life-threatening shock

These consensus guidelines were compiled by the Project Team of the Resuscitation Council (UK) and published in the Journal of Accident and Emergency Medicine in July 1999 [1]. The incidence of anaphylactic reactions appears to be increasing. The Resuscitation Council felt it necessary to publish these guidelines because of variations in published recommendations and in light of evidence that the treatment of anaphylaxis is often inadequate, with under-use of adrenaline and inappropriate use of intravenous (i.v.) (rather than intramuscular [i.m.]) adrenaline. The guidelines are the result of consensus opinion from experienced doctors as there have been no definitive clinical trials done.

Because of the lack of universally accepted definitions of anaphylactic and anaphylactoid reactions, and because they may both present with the same clinical manifestations, the document does not distinguish between them when considering emergency treatment.

Anaphylactic reactions vary in their severity and may progress at different rates. The clinical symptoms of anaphylaxis vary widely and this may lead to a difficulty in making an accurate diagnosis, particularly in children, with subsequent inappropriate treatment. Because future management may depend on an accurate diagnosis, it may be helpful to perform blood tests looking for specific immunoglobulin E (IgE) and mast cell tryptase. Blood samples are best taken 45 min after the onset of a suspected reaction.

The guidelines reiterate that, as always, it is vital to take a good history, including previous allergic reaction, and to make a thorough examination, particularly looking at the skin, pulse rate, blood pressure, upper airways and auscultating the chest. Peak flow should be recorded if possible.

Adrenaline works by reversing peripheral vasodilation, reducing laryngeal oedema, dilating airways, increasing myocardial contractility and suppressing leukotriene and histamine release. It works best when given early in the reaction and is very safe when given i.m. If given late it may fail to work, in which case the use of other drugs and volume expansion become more important.

Antihistamines should routinely be used in all anaphylactic reactions and are very safe. However, sole use without other intervention is unlikely to save lives.

Corticosteroids may take up to 6 h to exert their full effect even when given i.v. They may reduce the length of a reaction. There has been some concern in the past about using corticosteroids, but the document recommends that for safest practice, corticosteroids should be routinely used in all cases of severe anaphylaxis.

The guidelines show two algorithms for treating anaphylaxis, one for adults and one for children. The two are essentially the same, differing only in drug dosages and fluid volumes needed. These guidelines are as follows:

1. Lie patient in a comfortable position and give high-flow oxygen.
2. Administer i.m. adrenaline to patients with evidence of stridor, wheeze, respiratory distress or evidence of shock. A second dose of adrenaline may be given after 5 min in the absence of improvement or if there is deterioration, especially if the level of consciousness is dropping as a result of hypotension. In some cases improvement with adrenaline may not last long, in which case several doses may be needed. Some patients may have already had a dose of adrenaline from an Epipen™ or equivalent. These are usually 125 or 250 μg – the dose should be checked.
   i.v. adrenaline, even at a strength of 1:10 000 is dangerous and should not be used unless the patient has profound, life-threatening shock. If used, ECG monitoring is mandatory.
3. Administer antihistamine (chlorpheniramine) i.m. or by slow i.v. injection. Rapid administration may result in hypotension.
4. Administer hydrocortisone i.m. or by slow i.v. injection. It is particularly important to give this to asthmatics as they are at greater risk of severe or fatal anaphylaxis, especially if they have been on steroids.
5. If bronchospasm is severe and does not respond to the above drugs, inhaled salbutamol may be used.
6. If severe hypotension does not respond to this treatment volume expansion in the form of a crystalloid should be given. It may be necessary to give this rapidly or repeat the dose.

Some patients should be kept under observation for 8–24 h. This group should include those with slow onset reactions, those with severe asthma or who have had severe bronchospasm, and those with a previous history of biphasic reactions.

Following an anaphylactic reaction, patients should avoid any known allergen and be advised to wear an information tag such as a medicalert bracelet to inform bystanders in the future. The document recommends that there should be full investigation and follow-up at a specialist allergy clinic for those who have had severe reactions.

REFERENCES

1. Project Team of the Resuscitation Council (UK). Emergency Medical Treatment of Anaphylactic Reactions. *J Acc Emerg Med* 1999; **16**: 243–247.

Guidelines for Good Practice in the Management of Neonatal Respiratory Distress Syndrome

KEY POINTS

- Outlines best management, including prevention, of respiratory distress syndrome, using results of randomized controlled clinical trials where possible
- Surfactant is more effective when used prophylactically than as rescue therapy
- Ventilatory support should be used in babies requiring >50% oxygen
- High frequency ventilation is not established as superior to conventional ventilation

Issued in November 1999 by the British Association of Perinatal Medicine (BAPM), these guidelines outline the management of respiratory distress syndrome (RDS) [1]. They present the best evidence-based management practice in the prevention and treatment of RDS. The guidelines are also intended to provide a national standard of care for audit purposes.

The guidelines include extensive recommendations, which are targeted at obstetricians, for the antenatal management of infants at risk of RDS. For example, the use of antenatal steroids is recommended when delivery before 34 completed weeks is expected. These are more effective if given 48 h or more prior to delivery, but should be given even if delivery will occur sooner. Contra-indications to the use of steroids include chorioamnionitis and active maternal infection.

Effective resuscitation is key to the viability of preterm infants. Those who require more than minimal intervention should be intubated, and ventilated for transfer to the neonatal unit. Adrenaline (10 µg kg^{-1}) should be used for persisting bradycardia, given via the endotracheal route if intravenous access is not established. At least one dose should be given intravenously if the endotracheal dose is unsuccessful. A dose of 100 µg kg^{-1} can be tried if other doses are unsuccessful.

Surfactant therapy is recommended for all infants of less than 32 weeks gestation who require intubation. This is more effective as prophylaxis than as rescue therapy. The guidelines suggest that natural surfactant extracts are more effective than artificial surfactants. They also suggest that two doses of surfactant are thought to be more effective than a single dose; more than two doses has not been shown to be of greater benefit.

Continuous positive airway pressure (CPAP) or artificial ventilation should be used for babies who require ≥50% oxygen to maintain their oxygenation. Artificial ventilation should be considered when the arterial pH is below 7.25 and the arterial CO$_2$ tension (PaCO$_2$) is ≥7 kPa.

Conventional ventilation is discussed. The use of a high rate strategy is recommended as this results in a lower incidence of pneumothorax. The ventilator settings should be such that pressures are kept as low as possible to minimize barotrauma.

High frequency oscillation is yet to be shown to be superior to conventional ventilation. It is used as rescue therapy in most units, awaiting the results of the UK oscillation study (UKOS).

Arterial blood gas monitoring should be used in ventilated preterm infants. Hypocapnia should be avoided as it has detrimental effects on cerebral blood flow, with a resultant increase in periventricular leukomalacia. Ventilation should be adjusted to prevent the arterial pH falling below 7.25. The arterial O_2 tension (PaO_2) should be kept between 6 and 10 kPa, and, in general, the $PaCO_2$ above 5 kPa.

Hypotension should be treated as it is associated with an increase in cerebral haemorrhage and mortality. Volume expansion should be the first line of treatment. The second line treatment should be inotropic support. Dopamine is recommended at a dose of 10 μg kg^{-1} min^{-1}. If this is unsuccessful, dobutamine may be tried. Hydrocortisone and adrenaline may also be tried.

The guidelines recommend the use of steroids in infants who remain ventilator dependent at 2 weeks of age.

Preterm infants should be followed up in the community for at least 2 years post-discharge from hospital.

REFERENCE

1. Report of the Second Working Group of the British Association of Perinatal Medicine. *Guidelines for good practice in the management of neonatal respiratory distress syndrome.* BAPM Nov. 1999.

ETHICS

Guidelines for the Ethical Conduct of Medical Research Involving Children

KEY POINTS

Defines six principles which should govern the practice of research involving children:

* Research involving children is important. It should be conducted in an ethical manner
* Children have unique interests
* Research should only be done on children if comparable research on adults cannot answer the questions posed
* If the research does not directly benefit the child it is not necessarily unethical
* All proposals should be submitted to the local research ethics committee
* Consent should be obtained from children and parents as appropriate. Even with parental consent the agreement of school age children should be sought

Written by the British Paediatric Association (now the RCPCH) Ethics Committee and published in 1992, these guidelines are aimed at everyone involved in the planning, review and conduct of research involving children [1].

The six principles on which the guidelines are based are listed in the Key Points above.

The report stresses the importance of research involving children as a means of promoting child health and well being. Research projects need to be well designed and conducted. As children are at the start of their lives they are more likely to experience the most long lasting benefits or harm from research.

It is important that GPs and other staff involved with the child are fully informed about the research. Partnership, where research is carried out with children rather than on them should be encouraged. The declaration of Helsinki should be respected, i.e. concern for the interests of the child must prevail over those of science or society.

Adequate basic research should have been carried out to minimize the risks. Children should only be involved if research on adults is not feasible or would not answer the questions being asked. New procedures/treatments should first be tried on adults if possible, with time allowed to assess medium term effects.

Potential benefits/harm/costs should be carefully considered. If research does not directly benefit the child then only minimal risk is acceptable. Higher risks may be acceptable in serious illness and if the child is likely to benefit.

All proposals should be submitted to the local research ethics committee. However, everyone involved in research has some responsibility. Ethics is about good practice. Where children have significant understanding of the proposal and its implications it is their consent rather than their parents' which is needed. Where children are not able to fully understand, then the parents may consent (as long as it is not against the child's interests). If parental consent is given, then the agreement of school age children should also be sought.

These guidelines are designed to benefit children taking part in research, those who might be helped by research findings, and medical research itself.

REFERENCE

1. *Guidelines for the Ethical Conduct of Medical Research Involving Children*. London: Royal College of Paediatrics and Child Health. 1992.

Withholding or Withdrawing Life Saving Treatment in Children

KEY POINTS
- Provides guidelines for withholding or withdrawing care
- Defines five categories where this is acceptable
- Decisions should be made by senior staff
- Palliative care should always be offered
- Pain relief should always be maintained

These guidelines were published by the RCPCH in 1997 [1]. Following discussions by the House of Lord's Select Committee, the Ethics Advisory Committee of the BPA (now RCPCH) decided to explore the issues surrounding withdrawing and withholding life saving treatment in children. After 2 years of research involving parents, paediatricians, people of varied religion and nationality, ethicists and lawyers, this document was drawn up, taking into account existing law and the rights of a child.

It provides a framework which guides the difficult decision-making process necessary to withdraw or withhold life saving treatment in children. Five situations are described in which this may be appropriate:

- the brain dead child, where criteria are met in the usual way and there is agreement between two medical practitioners [2] (see also pages 84–85);
- the permanent vegetative state;
- the 'no chance' situation, where treatment simply delays death;
- the 'no purpose' situation, where the degree of physical or mental impairment caused by further treatment would be too much to expect the child to bear;
- the 'unbearable' situation, where either the child or family feel that, in view of their progressive and irreversible illness, further treatment is more than can be borne.

These categories do not include the withdrawal of palliative or terminal care.

Senior staff should make decisions about withdrawing or withholding of care and, in cases where insufficient information is available, the option of optimal life saving treatment should be taken in the first instance. At all times the welfare of the child must be paramount. Where possible children should be informed and involved in any decision making.

Neonatal practice is briefly mentioned. The already accepted practice of withholding resuscitation in babies who are extremely premature, or who have congenital abnormalities incompatible with life is upheld.

In babies who have proven profound brain damage (for example following severe birth asphyxia) and where the parents accept that the child is likely to be profoundly neurologically damaged, the practice of withdrawing artificial ventilation is also upheld.

Euthanasia is discussed and is expressly not approved of by the Ethics Advisory Committee of the RCPCH. However, a distinction is made between the justifiable use of a treatment which may incidentally hasten death, whilst relieving suffering, and deliberate euthanasia.

Changing management from life-sustaining treatment to palliation represents a change in beneficial aims, and does not constitute withdrawal of care. It is never permissible to withdraw procedures designed to alleviate pain or promote comfort.

Where treatment aimed at the alleviation or cure of a condition has been withdrawn, it is the duty of the clinical team to offer palliative care.

Where decisions are particularly difficult and there is dissent between health care professionals or parents, a second opinion should be sought. In rare cases the High Court may need to be consulted.

REFERENCES

1. *Withholding or Withdrawing Life Saving Treatment in Children.* London: Royal College of Paediatrics and Child Health. 1997.
2. *Diagnosis of Brain Stem Death in Infants and Children.* London: British Paediatric Association. 1991.

Diagnosis of Brain Stem Death in Infants and Children

KEY POINTS

- A diagnosis of brain stem death can only be made in children older than 2 months
- Diagnosis should be made by two experienced clinicians, at least one of whom is a consultant and one should not be involved in the child's care
- The use of electroencephalograms and other techniques such as Doppler measurements of cerebral blood flow are not a helpful part of diagnosis

This report was produced in 1991 by a working party of the British Paediatric Association (now the RCPCH) [1]. It examines the concept of brain stem death in children, and concludes that it is valid in children older than 2 months. The definition adopted is 'the irreversible loss of the capacity for consciousness, combined with the irreversible loss of the capacity to breathe'. In these cases it is established that asystole will inevitably follow despite continued support.

In children aged over 2 months of age, the adult criteria are used:

- the patient is comatose and requires mechanical ventilation for apnoea;
- there is an established cause for the coma;
- drugs (including paralysing agents) have been excluded as a cause;
- the child is not hypothermic;
- there is no endocrine or metabolic disturbance.

When these criteria are met the following tests of brain stem function are performed (on two separate occasions by two different clinicians) and must be absent:

- pupillary light reflexes;
- corneal reflex;
- vestibulo-ocular reflex;
- doll's eye reflex;
- response to pain in the area of the fifth cranial nerve;
- gag reflex;
- apnoea in the presence of a $PaCO_2$ >6.6 kPa and a normal PaO_2.

An important distinction is drawn between infants of less than 37 weeks gestation and older infants. In the premature infant there are great difficulties in establishing the diagnosis, as the criteria of apnoea and coma are frequently seen in babies who survive intact. There are no firm data about the development of gag and caloric reflexes in this age group. In view of these factors the concept of brain stem death is viewed as inappropriate in this group.

The most difficult group is children aged between 37 weeks gestation and 2 months post-term. In this group the criteria above may be met but the inevitability of asystole in these cases is not established. As such, the diagnosis of brain stem death is rarely certain.

The report touches on the withdrawal of care in cases where brain stem death is not established and this has been examined in greater depth by later reports [2] (see also pages 82–83).

REFERENCES

1. *Diagnosis of Brain Stem Death in Infants and Children*. London: British Paediatric Association. Nov. 1991.
2. *Withholding or Withdrawing Life Saving Treatment in Children*. London: Royal College of Paediatrics and Child Health. 1997.

The Genetic Testing of Children

KEY POINTS

- Predictive genetic testing is appropriate if the condition often occurs in childhood and if there is useful medical intervention
- Testing in children should not be done for adult onset disorders if there is no useful intervention
- Testing should generally not be performed in children to establish carrier status with a view to their future reproduction
- Further research is needed regarding social and psychological aspects of genetic testing

Published in the Journal Medical Genetics in 1994, this is the report of a working party of the Clinical Genetics Society (UK) [1]. Their aim was to examine the attitudes and practices of genetic testing of children amongst the medical profession. They assessed the extent to which testing takes place and under what circumstances it is justified, and then made recommendations for future practice.

Their methods were fourfold. They used a questionnaire survey and performed a prospective study over 12 months aimed at scientists, geneticists and paediatricians, to assess attitudes towards and extent of genetic testing of children. They also sent questionnaires to family support groups to gain information regarding parental views and attitudes. Finally, they looked at the legal aspects in order to establish what would legitimately be best for the child.

The two aspects of testing highlighted were predictive genetic testing of adult onset conditions and carrier testing (where the inherited disorder could have an effect on future children but not on the health of the carrier). They outlined potential disadvantages and advantages of testing.

Potential disadvantages:

- lack of confidentiality;
- future autonomy undermined;
- damage to self-esteem;
- distorted family perceptions of the child;
- discrimination in education, employment, insurance;
- difficulties establishing future relationships;
- breaches the policy of counselling pre/post testing.

Potential advantages:

- opportunity for child to adjust to circumstances;
- family openness;
- resolution of parental uncertainty;
- ensures test offered to all family;
- responsible attitude to future reproduction;
- able to plan education, career, housing, family finances.

Following the results of the surveys, the Working Party made a number of recommendations. These included that predictive testing in childhood is only acceptable if the condition being tested for occurs frequently in childhood and there is useful medical intervention. Where there is no useful intervention, testing should be deferred until the individual is adult enough to make their own informed decision, with an understanding of both the genetic and emotional consequences of any result. In these circumstances, it should be an obligation of the medical profession to offer testing when the child is older. Genetic testing of an 'at risk' child should not be a requirement prior to adoption placement.

The Working Party recommend further research into disorders where there is insufficient evidence to decide if a genetic diagnosis will be helpful in the medical management of a child who may not yet be affected. Further research is also needed to look at the social and psychological impact of genetic testing.

The Working Party highlighted the Children Act 1989 [2] (see also pages 4–5) which says that parents have a responsibility for the care of the child rather than rights over them, and that parents are expected to act in the best interests of the child. The implication of this is that children should not undergo genetic testing purely for the benefit of their parents (e.g. to relieve anxieties). Where a child is being considered for adoption, predictive testing should not occur any earlier than if the child had stayed in his/her original family. Discussion and counselling between adoption family and agency should help in these circumstances.

Finally, the working party stresses the need for family openness about the potential disorder throughout childhood to help in future autonomous decision making.

REFERENCES

1. Report of a Working Party of the Clinical Genetics Society (UK). The genetic testing of children. *J Med Gene* 1994; **31**: 785–797.
2. *The Children Act 1989*. The Staionary Office. 1989.

Commercial Sponsorship in the Royal College of Paediatrics and Child Health

KEY POINTS

- Provides guidance for members of the RCPCH, and for the RCPCH itself, on the acceptability of sponsorship and advertising
- The overriding concern is to act for the best interests of children
- Sponsorship from tobacco producers, arms manufacturers and exploiters of children is unacceptable
- Advises the setting up of a committee to monitor sponsorship in the College
- The College should invest only in companies that share its ethical outlook

Published by the Royal College of Paediatrics in 1999, this is the report of the Ethics Advisory Committee, chaired by Professor R. Harvey [1]. The Royal College has to balance the need for financial support for itself and its members with ensuring that it acts in the best interests of children at all times. A great diversity of opinion exists within the College concerning advertising and sponsorship. The report aims to draw together this opinion into a unified policy, whilst accepting that some individuals will have a differing approach.

The report examines the pros and cons of relationships with commercial companies. Some sources of advertising or sponsorship, such as tobacco manufacturers, can never be seen to be in the best interests of children. For other sources, such as the producers of medical equipment, there are usually no ethical concerns. A difficult middle ground exists around such items as breast milk substitutes.

Exploitation of children can occur in many ways. For example, advertisers may target children with products that are unsuitable for them, such as junk food. The availability of junk food is acceptable, but the targeting of children is less so. The College needs to consider each case carefully to ensure that there is no implicit support of child exploitation.

Breast milk substitutes pose a particular difficulty for the College. Opinions within the College differ widely. In developing countries breast milk substitutes cause many infant deaths due to the unavailability of hygienic preparation facilities. However, in some circumstances, such as maternal HIV infection, breast milk substitutes may be desirable. The College is committed to supporting UNICEF's baby friendly initiative. The College will not itself accept sponsorship from companies producing breast milk substitutes. However, individuals may be sponsored by producers of breast milk substitutes, and the college will accept advertisements from them.

The sponsorship of research is addressed by the report. Such research must be ethical, and those sponsored must be free to publish results regardless of their desirability to the sponsoring company.

REFERENCE

1. *Commercial Sponsorship in the Royal College of Paediatrics and Child Health.* London: Royal College of Paediatrics and Child Health. 1999.

EDUCATION, TRAINING AND MANPOWER

Hospital Doctors: Training for the Future (The Calman Report)

KEY POINTS

- Recommendations made to bring the UK into line with European directives
- Recognition that specialist training took too long in the UK
- Introduction of improved training programmes
- Single training grade (specialist registrar) to replace career registrar and senior registrar grades
- Introduction of Certificate of Completion of Specialist Training (CCST)

European directives made in 1975 proposed a mechanism for the mutual recognition of medical qualifications throughout the European Union (EU). The EU was threatening action as the UK was failing to meet these directives. Therefore, this report was produced in 1993 by a working party established by the Government. Its aim was to propose actions necessary to bring the UK into line with European directives on medical training. This would ensure mutual recognition of medical qualifications throughout the EU. It made a number of recommendations:

1. Shorten training programmes to enable most doctors to obtain their certificate of completion of specialist training (CCST) within 7 years of qualification.
2. CCST to be awarded by the GMC on the advice of the relevant Royal College as recognition that the doctor has been assessed as competent and eligible for consideration for appointment to a consultant post.
3. Medical Royal Colleges should propose specialist training programmes leading to the award of a UK CCST. Only experience fulfilling the standards set by the accrediting authority will be recognized towards the award of the UK CCST.
4. Registrar and senior registrar grades to be replaced by a combined higher training grade: specialist registrar.
5. Doctors awarded a UK CCST should be indicated as such on the Medical Register by the addition of 'CT' alongside their entry.

In addition to the main recommendations, the following points were also made by the working party:

- entry to training programmes must be competitive;
- the needs of overseas doctors must be accommodated;
- arrangements need to be flexible to meet the differing requirements of different specialities;
- all arrangements must comply with EU directives;
- proper account must be taken of those trainees aiming at a career in academic medicine. The interests of academic and research bodies must be protected;
- future consideration could be given to replacing all three current training grades (senior house officer, registrar and senior registrar) with a single specialist grade;

- manpower planning will be required to keep to a minimum the number of specialists who are in the 'gap' between the award of their CCST and appointment to a consultant post. This will involve regulation of the numbers in training, and an increase in consultant numbers;
- a doctor should be able to remain in a training post for a short period after the award of their CCST in order to obtain a consultant post. When an individual leaves having failed to obtain a consultant post there will be the option of retraining in another specialty, working outside the NHS until finding a consultant post, or obtaining a non-consultant career post;
- the shortening of specialist training may have a significant impact on workforce arrangements. It is likely to lead to an increase in the proportion of care provided by consultants;
- specialist registrar quotas are issued for each specialty by postgraduate deans.

Subsequently, the specialist registrar grade was introduced in 1995 and formally launched in 1996.

REFERENCE

1. *Hospital Doctors: Training for the Future. Report of the Working Group on Specialist Medical Training. The Calman Report.* Department of Health. 1993.

A Guide to Specialist Registrar Training – 'The Orange Book'

KEY POINTS

- Detailed explanation of Specialist Registrar training
- Defines LAT and LAS posts and entitlements
- Recommendations/requirements for a National Training Number application
- Flexible training conditions
- Detailed breakdown of record of in-training assessment
- Furthering education, i.e. study leave/research

The Guide to Specialist Training ('the orange book') is a 91-page document published in 1996 [1]. It follows on from 'Hospital Doctors: Training for the Future (The Calman Report)' published in 1993 [2]. Changes in training were designed to create a much more structured, organized but shorter training towards clinically independent consultants. Registrar and senior registrar posts being abolished in favour of a unified training grade, the specialist registrar (SpR) grade.

The guide does not focus on paediatrics in particular, but details the structure of all specialist registrar training, from the process of applying for a National Training Number to attaining the CCST. It also details the roles of various authorities involved in training. The Specialist Training Authority (STA) includes representatives of all the Royal Colleges, the Faculties of Public Health and Occupational Medicine, the GMC, two postgraduate deans, an NHS manager and a patient representative. Amongst other things, its role is to safeguard standards of postgraduate training in the UK and to ensure that colleges, faculties and joint training committees evaluate training programmes. It is also responsible for awarding CCSTs once doctors have completed the necessary higher specialist training programme successfully. The award of the CCST marks the end point of specialist training and indicates that a doctor has reached a standard high enough for independent practice as a consultant. When doctors are awarded the CCST they may apply to the GMC for entry onto the Specialist Register. Presence on this register is a legal requirement for a doctor taking up a consultant post.

The guide also introduced the national training number (NTN), a unique number issued to each doctor entering a specialist training programme and held as long as the trainee is in the SpR grade. NTNs are issued by postgraduate deans. The NTN has four main uses:

1. allows postgraduate deans to track trainee progression and plan future funding;
2. guarantees a place on the specialty training programme for as long as the number is held;
3. allows health departments to predict how many doctors can be accommodated on the training programme;
4. allows the Royal Colleges to plan future education and monitor current training programmes and trainees.

Overseas doctors with a right of indefinite residence may receive NTNs, those without the right will receive visiting training numbers (VTNs).

Where short-term appointments are available these may be considered as locum appointments for training (LAT) or for service (LAS). Only the LAT posts will be considered as counting towards the CCST. A CCST will not be awarded to doctors who have just had LAT posts, substantive placement in the SpR grade is necessary. It is possible to retain an NTN whilst doing research outside the NHS as long as certain conditions are fulfilled. The NTN is also kept if a trainee decides to undertake flexible training. It is possible in some circumstances for a trainee to move from one deanery to another, in which case a doctor does not have to compete for a place in the training programme. When moving deaneries, a new NTN must be issued. In rare circumstances it is possible for an NTN to be removed, e.g. if it is felt that a trainee cannot complete the programme. In these cases there are appeal procedures.

The guide has a section on appointment to the grade of SpR which gives details of the construction of an appointment committee and what each member is expected to do. Details are also given of short-listing and interview procedures. Feedback to candidates who have failed should be available.

There is also a section which explains flexible training in the SpR grade. Flexible training is intended to allow doctors who are unable to work full time, to train in line with full timers. Flexible training is allowed where there is a good reason to do so, such as family commitment. Regional postgraduate deans provide funding. Potential flexible trainees need to liaise as closely as possible with their regional postgraduate deans to ensure an appropriate training programme. Trainees may change from part-time to full-time training and vice versa. Educational programmes and CCST dates will need to be readjusted with any changes. Flexible trainees need to do a minimum of 50% of the full-time equivalent and are expected to do a pro rata share of the on-call commitment.

The section on overseas doctors looks at two groups: registrars without the right to indefinite stay, known as visiting specialist registrars (VSpR), and those who do have the right to indefinite stay, regardless of where they obtained their primary qualification, known as SpRs. In both cases, visiting training numbers (VTNs) can be awarded. The rights to training and immigration permits are discussed. Regional postgraduate deans can liase with the Home Office to enable VSpRs to extend their period of permit free training. The book strongly recommends that overseas doctors discuss their training requirements with the postgraduate dean of the area they wish to apply to, before actually applying for the grade. This will help ensure the most suitable appointment is made, as some applicants may not have enough time to reach the CCST and may be better off with a fixed-term training appointment (FTTA). Overseas doctors are also able to fill LAT and LAS posts. There is no 'quota' for overseas doctors. Posts specifically for VSpRs may be advertised if there are vacancies in the SpR grade. All overseas doctors need to be registered with the GMC.

All SpRs must have their progress formally assessed. The assessment must be structured, interactive and competency-based.

The record of in-training assessment (RITA) is completed annually by the post graduate deans office and the trainee. In itself it is not an assessment, but a record of annual reviews and progress through the grade. The records are forwarded to the relevant Royal College.

Various documentation is allowed as additional evidence of satisfactory progress including log books, case books, reports from supervisors, audit and research reports, results of tests and certificates of courses attended.

Satisfactory assessment, as dictated by measurement against defined criteria, allows progression to the next year of training. Where progress is not satisfactory, there are three levels of action which can follow:

1. Recommendation for targeted training: closer supervision with specific experiences to fill gaps. No delay of progress in training.
2. Recommendation for intensified supervision or repeat experience: usually when stage 1 has not worked.
3. Withdrawal from the programme: where progress has not been satisfactory despite actions and there is no reasonable chance of achieving it. Counselling for future career choices should be available.

There is an appeals procedure for trainees who wish to have decisions reviewed.

There are recommendations for the amount of study leave SpRs should be entitled to. There is also a section on research which essentially says that although encouraged, it is not a prerequisite to becoming a consultant. Time out for research should be carefully planned with appropriate career guidance. NTNs can be retained for up to 3 years of research.

Following completion of training, registrars should receive their CCST and apply for a consultant's job as soon as possible. This can take some time and a 6-month gap between finishing training and termination of employment in the SpR grade is allowed. If, despite trying hard, a consultant's post is not obtained, the postgraduate dean may allow a further contract in the SpR grade.

The sections regarding appointments to SpR training programmes and also the RITA include sample copies of application and assessment forms.

Overall, the document is aimed for use not only by specialist registrars, but in particular for those aspiring to be SpRs and those involved in the management of their training.

REFERENCES

1. *A Guide to Specialist Registrar Training*. Department of Health. 1996.
2. *Hospital Doctors: Training for the Future. Report of the Working Group on Specialist Medical Training. (The Calman Report)*. Department of Health. 1993.

Flexible Training in Paediatrics

KEY POINTS

- Each deanery should have a flexible training co-ordinator
- Due to increasing numbers of flexible trainees there will be problems finding placements, and more will need to job share
- Flexible trainees should be equal to full time trainees in every way except time commitment

This report was published by a working party of the RCPCH in 1999 [1]. Flexible training has increased significantly over the last decade and flexible trainees have become recognized as an important part of the workforce. Paediatrics has a large proportion of women doctors and subsequently has one of the highest levels of doctors working flexibly or in job-shares (an average 16% of paediatric SpRs in 1999 with up to 25% in some deaneries). This number is not expected to drop and may even increase in the future. There are problems encountered in flexible training and with the rise in numbers, the supernumerary scheme will not be able to cope. The working party set out to identify these problems and find ways of solving them.

Flexible training is open to doctors (male or female) with health problems or with family or other major commitments. There are many advantages of flexible training such as being able to continue training without the need for long career breaks to bring up children and the ability to tailor training to the needs of the trainee when in supernumerary posts. Paediatrics benefits as a whole by retaining experienced doctors through to consultant level and by having improved continuity of care (as trainees stay in posts for longer).

The working party drew up a list of real and perceived problems with flexible training. These include the fact that flexible trainees may be unemployed after appointment whilst awaiting funding, may not feel 'part of the team' and may not be given organizational tasks. They may be tied to one geographical area and so have difficulty getting training in their chosen specialty and may have particular difficulty obtaining a research grant. In addition, it may be difficult for trainees to attend educational activities, and supervision may be poor, especially in departments with large numbers of flexible trainees. Flexible trainees are often inflexible with regard to starting and finishing times, rota changes and doing extra hours for absent colleagues.

The working party has created three basic guidelines for flexible training programmes.

1. Flexible training should be equivalent to full-time training in all respects, so that there is single competition for job entry at SHO and SpR grade. Service and on-call commitments should be equivalent pro rata including weekends and paid time off after a night on call. There should be equal training opportunities, equal supervision, assessment, and educational opportunities and equal access to specialist training slots.

2. Departments should only take on as many flexible trainees as they can provide adequate training, supervision and service commitment for.
3. Flexible trainees should take responsibility for becoming part of their department and try to organize out of work commitments to give a degree of flexibility to working times, thereby allowing smooth running of the department.

The working party proposes that each deanery should appoint a flexible training coordinator to organize and run programmes for flexible trainees at SHO and SpR level. He will work with the paediatric regional advisor and the associate postgraduate dean.

The working party also proposes that training placements for flexible trainees could be identified. This can be achieved by getting departments to apply to take a flexible trainee and then gaining the approval of the STA and RCPCH for the post. In most cases only one flexible trainee at each level would be allowed per department. Consultants should not supervise more than two SpR trainees.

SHOs
For SHOs on the GP vocational training scheme (VTS), suitable placements would already have been identified. These SHOs should have an educational supervisor in the paediatric department and an overall supervisor within the VTS. For SHOs pursuing a career in paediatrics, suitable placements in pre-existing rotations and posts in neonates, general paediatrics and other specialties would be identified. SHOs should be able to transfer from full-time to part-time training for the remainder of their job, but will then need to apply for further jobs in open competition with full-time trainees.

SpRs
Doctors applying for SpR grade must do so in open competition and following appointment to the post may elect immediately or later to train flexibly. The trainee should liaise with the associate dean to arrange funding. Appointment to the post will be by the same system as full-time trainees, namely that the best candidates get first choice of available posts. If two trainees opt to train flexibly within the same department they may be expected to job-share. In some regions there is competition for year 4 and 5 posts, and in these cases flexible trainees will be expected to compete along side full-timers. Appraisal and assessment of flexible trainees will be the same as that for full-timers, including RITA assessment.

Job-sharing
With the increase in flexible trainee numbers, supernumerary posts are becoming harder to organize, and job-sharing is becoming more widely adopted as a solution to this problem. The working party looked at the job-share programme which has been successful in the North Thames region, and have made some guidelines for job-sharing. Selection of SpRs should be to the grade and not to any particular post. Rotations should be created so that posts are within easy geographical reach of each other. The flexible training co-ordinator and Calman Programme Director should identify training slots for flexible trainees, either stand-alone or job-share. Job-share should be considered where two trainees in the same department wish to train flexibly and could cover a substantive post between them. The associate dean would need to approve funding for two extra sessions, one for study leave and one for handover. In

some cases trainees may wish to do more than six sessions, in which case the dean would need to fund the extra sessions. If one part of the job-share leaves their post, the position converts to a supernumerary post and the space is filled with a full-time trainee. If one half of the job-share is ill or on annual leave it is the responsibility of the whole team to provide cover, and not just the other flexible trainee. The RCPCH will run a job-share register for trainees and consultants.

Inter-deanery transfer
Some flexible trainees will need to transfer deaneries. This must be for a good reason. In these circumstances trainees will retain their NTN until the next one is available in the new deanery. The postgraduate deans of both areas must approve the transfer.

On-call
There has been some variation in the on-call commitments undertaken by different flexible trainees. The working party clarifies that on-call should be equal pro rata to the rest of the team. This includes nights and weekends. The rota may be modified during breast-feeding, but this should mean being on-call for shorter periods rather than dropping out altogether. Trainees should try to be as flexible as possible regarding the rota and if contracted to, should also provide pro rata sick leave cover.

Additional Duty Hours (ADHs)
Since 1997, funding for ADHs has come from the employing trust and the postgraduate dean provides the rest of the funding for a flexible trainee. This may require negotiation between the trust and the deanery on behalf of the trainee. This way of funding may be re-examined by the NHS Executive in the future.

NTNs
Flexible trainees retain their NTNs for several years longer than their full-time counterparts. This has resulted in a mismatch between the anticipated number of consultant vacancies and NTNs required by trainees. There is a proposal that NTNs could be linked to the anticipated CCST date, rather than start date, thereby freeing up more numbers for full-time trainees. However, there is a planned reduction in the number of NTNs available over the next few years.

Research
All trainees should have the opportunity of taking part in research at some point in their careers. This is a necessity for those who wish to have an academic career and desirable in those intending to practice as tertiary specialists. Flexible trainees are in the fortunate position of being able to undertake longer term projects and should be actively encouraged to do this. Where time is spent on a research programme, it should be on research appropriate to the trainees intended career. It should be well supervised and have the support of the postgraduate dean and regional advisor.

Specialty paediatrics
Flexible trainees wishing to become tertiary specialists should be given any necessary help and advice. They should liaise with local specialists, the flexible training advisor and regional advisor to create a training programme. As before, appointment will be by the same process as for full-timers.

Part-time consultant posts

With increasing numbers of junior staff working part-time it is anticipated that there will need to be more part-time consultant posts available. The working party recommends that the RCPCH support the creation of part-time posts in every department. This would also enable older consultants to drop some sessions before retiring.

REFERENCES

1. Report of a Working Party. *Flexible training in paediatrics*. London: Royal College of Paediatrics and Child Health. 1999.

FURTHER READING

1. *Family Friendly Working Practices*. London: Royal College of Paediatrics and Child Health. 1999.
2. *Flexible Training in Paediatrics*. RCPCH leaflet for trainees. London: Royal College of Paediatrics and Child Health. 1999.

The Doctors' Tale – The Work of Hospital Doctors in England and Wales

KEY POINTS

- Describes demographics, skill mix and deployment of hospital doctors
- Describes the ways in which doctors work and train
- Identifies problem areas and suggests solutions

This report was published by the Audit Commission in 1995 [1].

The Audit Commission was set up to review the economy, efficiency and effectiveness of services provided by the NHS. It studies different areas every year. In 1995 it studied hospital medical staffing on the basis that doctors account for approximately 14% of an acute hospital's annual budget, and the fact that doctors everywhere are being affected by major changes in healthcare. These changes include an increasingly autonomous hospital management, a more structured approach to medical training and Government policy which aims to reduce doctors' working hours. The aim of the report was to identify problem areas in the ways doctors work, train and interact with the rest of the hospital, and, wherever possible, to suggest solutions.

Chapter 1 describes the demographics of hospital doctors in 1995. At this time there were approximately 55 000 hospital doctors in England and Wales. After SHO training about 42% of doctors remain in hospital medicine, 33% become GPs and the rest are divided into academic medicine, other NHS medicine, non-NHS medicine and very few leave medicine altogether. In paediatrics, the ratio of trainees to consultants was 2.2:1 (compared with 1.8:1 in general medicine and 1.4:1 in general surgery). The increasing demand on health service provision has necessitated an increase in the number of doctors and a change in working pattern. In 1987 this led to three basic Government initiatives: 'Achieving a Balance' which aimed to increase the number of career grade doctors, 'The New Deal' which aimed to reduce doctors' working hours, and the 'Calman Report' (see also pages 92–93) which aimed to bring the training of UK doctors into line with those in the rest of the EU by reducing the length of time taken to reach consultant grade. In the year 2000 these remain controversial areas with many targets still not being met.

Chapter 2 looks at the skill mix and deployment of doctors. Despite the fact that more than 50% of people entering medicine are women, the more senior posts are predominantly filled by men. This is due to unnecessarily onerous on-call requirements, poor career advice and lack of suitable part-time career posts. An audit of doctors' activities during the day and night showed that many tasks inappropriate to the level of skill and training of doctors were being carried out by junior doctors, such as giving i.v. drugs and collecting equipment from other wards. Another audit showed that a large number of surgical SHOs were operating largely unsupervised for most of their operations, and that as many as 20% of outpatient clinics in general medicine and surgery were run by SHOs. This inadequate supervision has implications for training as well as patient care. The Audit Commission recommend that the allocation of appropriate tasks to junior doctors should be clarified and that supervision should be improved with access to a consultant in all settings and at all times. The commission also advocates the greater use of shift work in order that the number and skills of doctors available at a given time are appropriate for the number and type of patients being seen. They recognize that this may interfere with continuity of care. They also recommend the provision of posts which are equally accessible to the growing number of doctors with family commitments.

Chapter 3 looks at the contribution of consultants to the health service, their commitments and job plans. Historically consultants have been fairly free to set their own agendas. However, it has become increasingly obvious that their hospital commitments need to be formalized as a job plan which specifies exactly what is expected on an individual basis. Whole-time and maximum part-time consultants are employed for 11 notional half days of which 5–7 sessions should be allocated to fixed commitments. An audit of 60 consultants showed that there is, in fact, a wide variation in the level of fixed commitments which is not explained by their on-call duties. After adjusting for case complexity it is the number of fixed commitments attended rather than the speed of a consultants work which has the major effect on the amount of work done. An analysis of surgical work showed that some consultants do significantly more work than others, mainly because they work for longer hours (by attending more sessions) and less so because they work faster. The effect of private practice is surmised as a reason for the variation in individuals' contributions. Consultants employed on whole time contracts are not supposed to earn the equivalent of more than 10% of their gross NHS salary from private practice. An audit showed that for most consultants the amount of work done privately was not related to the amount of work done for the NHS. However, the 25% of consultants doing the most private work do significantly less NHS work than their colleagues. The Audit Commission recommend that all consultants should have job plans which are 'comprehensive, consistent, monitored and regularly reviewed'.

Chapter 4 looks at postgraduate training and continuing professional development. There are four basic guidelines drawn up by the GMC in conjunction with the Royal Colleges. These are that there should be proper induction training at the beginning of a post, an educational supervisor should be appointed, a training programme specific to the trainee should be drawn up and there should be proper assessment and appraisal. In 1995, to a large extent, these guidelines were not being adhered to locally. The Audit Commission recognizes that there needs to be a balance between service commitments and training for doctors, but points out that the need for continuing education is now generally accepted. An audit of consultants and their juniors showed large inconsistencies with consultants feeling that they were meeting many of the guidelines and the junior doctors feeling that very few were being met. The Audit Commission makes a number of recommendations including the appointment of a specific consultant within each directorate to be responsible for training policy and the appointment of a personal educational supervisor for each trainee. This should allow a more structured and individual approach to training. The Commission also recommend a 5% increase in the number of part-time training posts by the year 2000. In 1995 consultants and staff grade doctors had very variable access to study leave and funds for continuing medical education (CME). The Audit Commission recommends that each trust put into place policies for CME as part of their training strategy and that Royal Colleges should set definite training standards at all levels.

Chapter 5 provides a framework on which to implement some of the changes recommended. The basis is that as rules about doctors' working patterns are implemented there will be less of a need for the individual colleges to control posts and more control will fall into the hands of the trusts. In order to implement the recommendations made throughout the report there will need to be national controls (i.e. DoH guidelines), incentives for doctors to take part in the changes (i.e. pay awards and better hours deals) and better working relationships between doctors and managers.

The report recommends that NHS trusts retain the freedom to employ new consultants on whatever terms and conditions they wish, within the national terms and conditions of service. This allows local pay incentives to attract doctors to particular posts. There is a national system of performance awards for consultants. These are the distinction awards. Decisions to make awards A+, A and B are made at national level, and regionally for C awards. The values vary from 20% basic salary for C awards to 100% for A+ and are subject to a 5-yearly review. There is central funding for the top pay awards but local awards come out of local budgets and to this end the Audit Commission recognizes that in view of the large sums of money involved (£104 million in 1993/4), trust managers should 'have an unconditional veto on local awards'.

The Audit Commission recognizes the need for clinicians to play a more active part in the management of their work and of the trusts. It recommends that clinical directors take a lead role in staffing issues including implementing the changes recommended in this report. The trust board, chief executive and clinical directors all need to work together to agree strategies and implement the changes.

REFERENCES

1. The Audit Commission. *The Doctors' Tale, The Work of Hospital Doctors in England and Wales.* The Stationary Office. 1995.

FURTHER READING

1. *The Medical Workforce in Paediatrics and Child Health. 1995–1997.* London: Royal College of Paediatrics and Child Health. June 1998. (see also pages 104–105).

The Medical Workforce in Paediatrics and Child Health 1995–1997

KEY POINTS

- Describes paediatric workforce census data from 1995 and 1996
- Describes the speciality breakdown of England's paediatric consultants
- Predicts the need for paediatric consultant post expansion
- Describes the planned reduction in specialist registrar numbers
- Predicts an over supply of MRCP graduates for specialist registrar posts
- Forecasts an excess of trainees for some subspecialty groups

This report was produced in 1998 by the Royal College to look at the composition of the medical workforce in paediatrics [1]. This in turn allowed the prediction of future consultant post availability and also the availability of suitably qualified trainees to fill these posts.

The introduction of Calman training with the resultant reduction in junior doctor's hours has implications for the workload placed upon consultants. These were studied in the production of this report.

The paediatric medical workforce was described by a census carried out by British Paediatric Association (BPA) tutors in 1995. This described the name, grade and workplace of all doctors in paediatrics. A further census of paediatric consultants was performed in 1996, looking at specialty and planned retirement date. The numbers of higher specialist trainees were also examined through the data held by regional advisors and deans.

This data showed that there had been a steady increase in hospital consultant numbers from 1988 to 1996, of approximately 10% per annum. Over the same time interval registrar numbers had doubled, but the senior SHO grade had reduced considerably. In the community, consultant numbers had increased dramatically with a marked reduction in the numbers of senior clinical medical officers and clinical medical officers (SCMOs and CMOs, respectively).

The age distribution of consultants was examined and the majority were aged between 45 and 55 years. Overall, 62% of consultants were male.

Through looking at planned retirements, the expected completion of training by trainees, and potential expansion of consultant numbers, the report modelled the likely future need for specialist registrars. This showed that once the planned expansion of registrars was complete, there would then need to be a reduction in numbers to avoid massive over supply. This in turn would result in an over supply of trainees with the MRCP (now MRCPCH) compared to available specialist registrar posts. The planned reduction of 50 specialist registrar posts per annum has recently been increased to 100 posts per annum.

The career intentions of those in the registrar grade were examined, though the response rate was low. Through looking at this information and the potential availability of consultant appointments, the report predicts an over supply of trainees in both paediatric oncology and neurology.

Finally, the report examines the likely future changes in consultant working patterns, predicting that future services are more likely to be consultant led or provided. The increase in female consultant numbers is likely to increase the numbers of consultants working flexibly, and hence increase consultant numbers.

REFERENCES

1. *The Medical Workforce in Paediatrics and Child Health. 1995–1997.* London: Royal College of Paediatrics and Child Health. June 1998.
2. The Audit Commission. *The Doctors' Tale, The Work of Hospital Doctors in England and Wales.* The Stationary Office. 1995.

Continuing Medical Education for Career Grade Paediatricians

KEY POINTS

- Accumulate 250 CME credits over 5 years evenly spread between internal and external CME (ICME and ECME) credits
- Annual appraisal to formulate personal development plan
- Maintain a portfolio of evidence of CME activity
- Five categories of CME activity according to venue and level of organization

This was published by the RCPCH in 1997 [1].

There has always been a need for the continuing medical education (CME) of all practising consultants and other non-training career grades of staff (associate specialists, clinical medical officers and staff grades). Paediatricians have addressed this by attending meetings, courses, conferences, etc., and reading journals. Over the past 10 years or more there has been an increased interest in CME, particularly in the light of heightened public awareness, the need for patients to have confidence in their doctors and the advent of clinical governance. As a result of this CME has become more formalized. In 1994, the British Paediatric Association (now the RCPCH) set up a pilot scheme for CME. This proved successful and the national scheme for CME was implemented in 1996 for all career grade RCPCH members. It is now estimated that 80% of hospital doctors are taking part. Since January 2000 there are three separate requirements:

1. Accumulate 250 CME credits over 5 years by taking part in appropriate educational activities. These should be divided equally into internal and external continuing medical education (ICME and ECME, respectively), and should be spaced evenly over the 5 year period, i.e. 50 CME credits per year.
2. Undertake annual appraisal to plan the year's CME activity in advance. This personal development plan should be agreed by the employer and adequate resources provided to execute it.
3. Maintain a portfolio of evidence of CME activity.

Five categories of CME activity have been defined according to venue and level of organization. These are:

1 **International and National Meetings:** Meetings organized under the auspices of the RCPCH; Meetings organized by the Royal Colleges, the Royal Society of Medicine and other national and international bodies involved in the care and health of children; International clinical or scientific meetings; Research and research society meetings.
2 **Regional Meetings**
3 **Local Meetings**

4 **Self-directed Activities:** Prepared teaching packages/distance learning courses; Preparation of new postgraduate lectures; Medical postgraduate examining.
5 **Courses/Apprenticeship Activities:** Specific courses; Apprenticeship courses, e.g. learning a new technique, updating clinical management skills, attendance at specialist clinics; Learning from colleagues in inpatient/outpatient/community situations.

Some activities which do not count as CME credits include reading journals, delivery/preparation of presentations, undergraduate teaching, writing books and attending committees.

Each region has a regional adviser whose roles include approval of internal and external CME activities and the promotion of appropriate CME activities within the region.

The phrase continuing medical education (CME) has now been replaced by continuing professional development (CPD) in recognition of the fact that medical education is only one part of a clinician's professional development.

REFERENCE

1. *Continuing Medical Education for Career Grade Paediatricians.* London: Royal College of Paediatrics and Child Health. 1997.

DEVELOPMENT OF CHILDREN'S SERVICES

Paediatric Services within the Community for the New Millennium

KEY POINTS

- Outlines the essential tasks of community services
- Examines methods of delivery in the context of the governments plans for 'the new NHS'
- Makes broad recommendations for the shape of future community services

The structure and function of community paediatric services is undergoing change, principally driven by changes in government policy. This report, produced by a working party of the RCPCH in 1999, looks at the possible future directions for the provision of community paediatric services [1].

The RCPCH have previously outlined their recommended roles of community paediatric services. This report briefly summarizes those recommendations, identifying the essential tasks of a community service as:

- child protection;
- adoption and fostering;
- care of children with disabilities;
- educational medicine;
- specialist immunization services, and specialist clinics, such as enuresis, etc.;
- child health surveillance.

The future structure for the provision of community paediatric services remains uncertain. The creation of primary care groups, and later primary care trusts, will probably change the current pattern of delivery. The report is concerned that this will result in fragmentation of community child health provision to the point where the required critical mass for a safe and effective service is no longer attained.

The report also suggests that breaking up of existing provision must be avoided and recommends that the PCGs should commission services from community trusts. This can be achieved through integrated planning of service provision, both locally and nationally. Whilst community services are delivered in the primary care setting, their provision is more specialized than is usual for primary care, and as such primary care groups are unlikely to be the best providers.

To maintain efficient community paediatric services it may be necessary for there to be some amalgamation of community and acute paediatric services.

Links with community mental health services are discussed. There is an overlap between mental health and community paediatric services in areas such as behavioural problems. These problems should be managed in partnership between the two specialties.

The report concludes that whilst change is inevitable, the focus must be upon extension of existing services when they are functioning well. In the future, specialist care should continue to be provided by paediatricians, child mental health services and the allied professionals separate from primary care groups and trusts.

REFERENCE

1. *Paediatric Services Within the Community for the New Millennium.* London: Royal College of Paediatrics and Child Health. March 1999.

FURTHER READING

1. Report of a Working Party. *The Essentials of Effective Community Health Services for Children and Young People.* London: Royal College of Paediatrics and Child Health. November 1997.

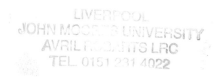

Accident and Emergency Services for Children

KEY POINTS
- Separate facilities for children and adult patients
- Only hospitals with paediatric inpatient services should accept children
- At least one registered children's nurse should be on duty at all times
- Trusts must recruit an A & E consultant with paediatric training
- A consultant paediatrician should be designated to liaise with A&E
- A&E medicine, primary care and paediatrics must collaborate nationally and locally

This report was produced in 1999 by a multidisciplinary working party convened by the RCPCH [1]. Its purpose was to make recommendations for the provision of accident and emergency services for children based on advice from the DoH, professional organizations and relevant consumer groups. Current arrangements for A&E services for children were reviewed and recommendations for future provision of services and training were made.

About 3.5 million children attend A&E departments in the UK each year. Health authorities and trusts have been slow to implement previous recommendations on staffing and facilities particularly in district general hospitals.

This report makes specific recommendations on facilities, function, staffing and inter agency cooperation within A&E departments.

Facilities must include separate play/waiting areas, treatment rooms, resuscitation beds and observation beds for children. Observation beds should be staffed by at least one registered children's nurse. A play specialist should supervise the provision of play facilities and decoration.

Children with other than minor injuries should, wherever possible, be directed to a hospital with inpatient paediatric services and a plan should be in place for this. All children should be triaged using a National Triage Scale, with immediate assessment of children carried into the department. A children's pain assessment tool should be used if appropriate.

Recommendations are made concerning the staffing of A&E departments, and the training of staff. A children's nurse trained in paediatric life support should be on duty at all times. Doctors should be advanced paediatric life support (APLS) trained. There should be a paediatric trained A&E consultant in each department, who should liaise with a designated paediatrician.

All A&E staff should be trained in child protection. Every A&E department must have a written child protection plan and timely access to the child protection register. A system of auditing frequent attendees should be in place, so that they are seen by a senior A&E doctor.

The child's GP and health visitor should be informed of every attendance.

Effective health promotion information and advice must be available. Each department should have a written policy for the support of bereaved families.

REFERENCE

1. Report of a Multidisciplinary Working Party. *Accident and Emergency Services for Children.* London: Royal College of Paediatrics and Child Health. June 1999.

Ambulatory Paediatric Services in the UK

KEY POINTS
- Ambulatory care represents a philosophy rather than a sub-specialty
- Delivery of specialist care in the community should occur wherever possible
- Ambulatory care aims to minimize hospital admissions and lengths of stay

This is the report of a working party published by the RCPCH in 1998 [1] in order to clarify the meaning of the term 'ambulatory care' when used in service planning and the appointment of consultants.

The report looks at British models of care and considers changes in acute morbidity which are likely to occur over the next two decades.

The term 'ambulatory care' is widely used with different meanings. Over the last few years in the UK it has come to mean services which mainly involve the acute or urgent specialist assessment of children admitted to hospital only briefly, if at all, for observation. They are usually referred by GPs or A&E departments and as such ambulatory care is not a primary health care service.

The working party looked at changes likely to occur in acute paediatric morbidity over the next 20 years. They felt that the development of vaccines against rotavirus, respiratory syncitial virus (RSV) and meningococcal disease would significantly reduce admission rates. Admission rates should also be reduced through better asthma prophylaxis and the use of home care nursing teams. However, the report also recognized that the number of children with chronic disability is rising.

The working party looked at the concept of ambulatory paediatrics as a separate sub-specialty but decided that it is a style of working which is adopted by most paediatricians working in secondary or tertiary care. Thus, they describe it as a philosophy which lies behind the provision of a service for children at home. The working party felt that the provision of paediatric services should take into account both the geographic and the demographic characteristics of the area.

The working party looked at the titles given to consultant paediatricians and the implications this has for ambulatory paediatrics. They felt that each consultant, irrespective of title, would need to take a degree of responsibility for community child health and that it would be a good idea for one consultant to take responsibility for ambulatory paediatric assessment. They recognize that this may be difficult in large tertiary centres.

The working party point out the importance of audit, monitoring and research in view of the evolving nature of ambulatory paediatrics. They recommend the collection of data on acute contacts with children who are not admitted or who receive care in a short stay unit. They specify that children admitted to short stay observation units should have the same data collected as those admitted more conventionally. They suggest that any follow up of these children could be done either by community children's nurses at home or by clinicians in a clinic set aside for this purpose.

Following these discussions, the RCPCH Council endorsed some agreements in 1997, including the following:

- ambulatory care is a philosophy lying behind provision of care and not a sub-specialty of paediatrics;
- paediatric and child health services should provide care without hospital admission whenever possible. When admission is needed, duration should be reduced to a minimum;
- the RCPCH should not support the use of the term ambulatory in consultant post titles, although it can be used as part of a job description.

REFERENCE

1. *Ambulatory Paediatric Services in the UK*. London: Royal College of Paediatrics and Child Health. 1998.

Children's Surgical Services

KEY POINTS

- Half of all paediatric admissions are for surgical care
- The majority of paediatric surgery comes within general surgical practice
- Surgery for complex or rare conditions should be done in specialist centres
- Children should not be treated on adult wards
- Day case surgery should be used where possible

Produced in 1996, this report was the result of an ad hoc committee set up by the RCPCH [1]. A previous report on surgery in children had failed to examine the full range of surgical specialities [2].

The report first makes several general recommendations for paediatric surgical practice. There are individual position statements produced by the colleges and specialist associations involved in surgery.

The report recommends that each hospital operating on children should have an appropriately trained consultant surgeon responsible for paediatric surgery. There should be a sufficient paediatric surgical workload to maintain his skills. Similarly, there should be a suitably trained consultant anaesthetist responsible for paediatric anaesthesia who also has an adequate paediatric workload to maintain his skills.

Anaesthesia in children under 5 years of age should be performed, or directly supervised, by a suitably experienced consultant anaesthetist.

Children should be transferred to specialist centres when suitably experienced staff are unavailable.

For children with rare or complex surgical conditions, surgery should be performed in specialist centres where there are paediatric high dependency facilities with access to paediatric intensive care.

Day case surgery should be used wherever possible.

The report recommends that paediatric surgery should only be performed in hospitals with a fully staffed paediatric department.

REFERENCES

1. Report of an ad hoc Multidisciplinary Children's Surgical Liaison Group. *Children's Surgical Services*. London: Royal College of Paediatrics and Child Health. Dec. 1996.
2. *The Transfer of Infants and Children for Surgery*. London: British Paediatric Association, Feb. 1993.

Surgical Services for the Newborn

KEY POINTS

- Neonates requiring surgery should be treated in regional neonatal surgical centres
- These centres should have full facilities for the care of the surgical neonate
- Neonatal surgical units should have a minimum of four consultant surgeons and a paediatric urologist
- A foetus with suspected major congenital malformation should be delivered in a hospital with a paediatric surgical unit

This report was first produced by the Royal College of Surgeons of England and the British Association of Paediatric Surgeons in 1992 in answer to the needs identified in the National Confidential Enquiry into Peri-Operative Deaths [1]. This update, published in 1999, builds upon the original report and extends its recommendations [2].

The report identifies the changing surgical needs of the neonatal population due to improved antenatal screening. There is less need for surgery for abnormalities of the central nervous system (e.g. spina bifida). There has been an increase in the surgical problems of the premature neonate such as necrotizing enterocolitis and inguinal hernia, brought about by the increased survival of extremely low birth weight infants.

With referral to regional neonatal units, the report identifies a reduction in mortality for oesophageal atresia and tracheo-oesophageal fistula. This reduction in mortality through the use of regional units leads to the recommendation that all neonatal surgery should be carried out in such units. For conditions such as congenital diaphragmatic hernia, it recognizes that management has changed and that immediate surgery is no longer standard practice.

The report recognizes that a wide range of specialities are needed for the care of the surgical neonate, and again it is suggested that this is best realized in regional centres. To achieve the critical mass required these units should have a minimum of 12 cots of which half should be for intensive care.

Nursing requirements are addressed and staffing levels suggested. The training requirements for neonatal nurses in surgical units are addressed.

Requirements for neonatal anaesthesia are also discussed, both with regard to training and service. It is recommended that there should be continuous cover by suitably experienced consultant anaesthetists.

The report addresses the transport needs for patients referred to regional units. For a foetus with suspected major congenital malformation the report recommends that transfer should, where possible, be done *in utero*. This can either be performed by the surgical unit or the referring hospital according to locally agreed protocols. The parents of a delivered infant also require transfer to the regional centre to further the development of the parent–child bond.

The report concludes with a useful table giving the incidences of neonatal surgical conditions.

REFERENCES

1. Campling EA, Devlin HB, Lunn JN. *The Report of the National Confidential Enquiry into Perioperative Deaths 1989*. London: National Confidential Enquiry into Peri-operative Deaths (NCEPOD). 1990.
2. *Surgical Services for the Newborn. Commission on the Provision of Surgical Services*. British Association of Paediatric Surgeons and The Royal College of Surgeons of England. June 1999.

A Guide to the Development of Children's Palliative Care Services

KEY POINTS

- Paediatric palliative care services in the UK are inadequate
- Palliative care is needed for children with long-term life-limiting conditions as well as those with a short time left to live
- The prevalence of children needing palliative care is approximately 1/1000
- Regional coordinated palliative care services need to be set up

This is the report of a joint working party of the Association of Children with Life-threatening or Terminal Conditions and Their Families (ACT) and the RCPCH published in 1997 [1]. The working party was set up in light of the fact that palliative care services for children in the UK are few and far between. The aim of the report is to clarify the needs of children with life limiting conditions who are likely to die in childhood, or soon after, including those with severe disabling conditions, e.g. severe cerebral palsy, to provide recommendations to purchasers on the services which should be provided to meet these needs, and to advise on the training and staffing needed for these services.

For the purposes of the report, life-limiting conditions are divided into four broad groups:

- conditions for which curative treatment is theoretically possible but where palliative care may be necessary in times of prognostic uncertainty or when treatment fails, e.g. cancer, irreversible organ failure;
- conditions where there may be long and intensive periods of treatment aimed at prolonging life but where childhood or early adult death is likely, e.g. cystic fibrosis;
- conditions which are progressive over many years where there is no treatment option other than palliative care, e.g. Batten's disease;
- conditions with severe neurological disability whose sequelae may lead to further health complications including sudden deterioration, e.g. severe cerebral palsy.

The number of children dying is small compared to the number of adults dying. In 1997 data suggests that in a district with 50 000 children, five each year are likely to die from progressive conditions for which palliative care is appropriate (two of these from cancer, one from heart disease and two from other life-limiting conditions) and a further 50 are likely to have a life-limiting condition for which palliative care is appropriate, for half of whom this need is likely to be substantial. Currently the most comprehensive services provided are for those children with malignancies, but for children with other life-limiting conditions the service provision is much more limited. In 1997 there was only one paediatric palliative care consultant in the UK, most families had infrequent and irregular contact with the consultant involved in their child's care, there were a small number of clinical nurse specialists working mainly from tertiary referral centres, thus limiting the number of children easily reached, and the small number of community children's nursing services available were seriously under resourced. The onus often falls on parents and GPs to look after children with long term conditions, but this is difficult and many of the conditions are very rare.

In 1997 there were 11 children's hospices (funded by the private sector) providing respite care for children and their families. A further 11 were in the planning stage. By 2002 all areas of the country should have reasonable access to a children's hospice. A small amount of paediatric palliative care is provided by the adult palliative care services. This may help bridge the gap in service provision for teenagers.

The report lays out some principles to guide purchasers and providers of palliative care. These include the need for a service which cooperates with other departments, and which is child/family centred and flexible depending on the needs of the individual child and family. There should be a key worker for each child to coordinate and plan service provision. There should be continuity of care between hospital and the community and home, and in the transition to adult services where appropriate. Staff working with these children should be appropriately qualified and have training in palliative care. Purchasers also need to take into account the rights of a child as defined in the Children Act (see also pages 4–5), the UN Convention on the Rights of a Child [2] (see also pages 48–49), The Patients' Charter, The Welfare of Children and Young People in Hospital and the Education Act [3]. The report points out that in order to provide adequate local services there needs to be much better morbidity data.

There has been a significant amount of research done on the needs of families with a child with a life-limiting condition which have resulted in some key recommendations [4]. These include the need for families to have simple written information and opportunities for questions and discussion. Information regarding financial and other non-statutory help should be made available at an early stage. Families need access to 24 h medical/nursing advice and support, especially at the time around death when symptoms may change quickly. Parents should be allowed to choose where their child dies and services should be provided to allow this. Following death practical information should be provided on what needs to be done next. Each district should have a senior paediatrician to coordinate a multidisciplinary network of children's palliative care. The services of the paramedical professionals, e.g. occupational therapists, should be provided in accessible central locations. Each family should have an identified local consultant who knows their child's condition. Planned, regular respite care is needed to give carers breathing space and should be provided more widely. The report recommends that psychological and emotional support, including a bereavement support service should be provided for the whole family. Some families may have inherited conditions and a genetic service should therefore be available to them. The report recognizes the additional burden put on parents trying to obtain all the necessary medication and equipment and recommends the coordination of this through a central system. Children with palliative care needs often spend significant proportions of their lives undergoing treatments with the detrimental effect of losing play and education time. It is important that this is recognized and that every effort is made to normalize their day to day living as much as possible.

There is a section of the report aimed at providers of health care services which essentially reiterates the need for establishing databases of these children and the need for multidisciplinary teams, within which there should be a core group who meet regularly to discuss palliative care referrals and other issues. This core group could then act as a resource to other professionals involved. The report also recommends the existence of an overall district coordinator of palliative care who should be an experienced health care professional with enough time to perform this duty.

The last section of the report discusses research and training in palliative care. There has been relatively little research done in paediatric palliative care which makes evidence-based medicine difficult in this field. The report makes recommendations as to areas where research is needed. These include outcome measures and the epidemiology of life threatening conditions.

The report suggests that every one who comes into contact with terminally ill children should be trained in communication skills. For doctors there is no formal accredited training for paediatric palliative care. The report suggests that in each region there could be a single paediatric consultant with palliative care as a full or part time academic interest. This would enable the creation of training posts. Although there are training courses for nurses which include an element of palliative care there are no specific paediatric care courses. These are urgently needed. Specific short courses need to be available for other people looking after these sick children, e.g. those offering short-term respite care. There is one children's hospice which offers one day workshops.

The impact on the staff working with terminally ill children should not be forgotten. They need regular and frequent support and access to people who can help with stress management. Supervision for these professionals should be written into their job descriptions.

REFERENCES

1. *A Guide to the Development of Children's Palliative Care Services*. A joint working party of ACT and the RCPCH. London: Royal College of Paediatrics and Child Health. 1997.
2. *The UN Convention on the Rights of the Child*. UNICEF, 1989.
3. *The Education Act*. The Stationary Office, 1996.
4. While A, Citrone C, Cornish J. *The Welfare of Children and Young People in Hospital*. 1996. *A study of the needs and provisions for families caring for children with life-limiting incurable disorders*. Department of Nursing Studies, King's College, London.

Guidance for Services for Children and Young People with Brain and Spinal Tumours

KEY POINTS

- Twenty-five per cent of childhood cancers are CNS tumours
- About 35% of children with CNS tumours are not receiving care from specialist centres
- Provides guidelines for a national framework of care for children with CNS tumours
- Age-specific care to be concentrated in centres with full range of necessary treatment and support facilities
- Emphasis on multidisciplinary teams
- Registration with UKCCSG to be increased, allowing better data collection
- Research and clinical trials to be encouraged
- Better coordination of services may improve morbidity and mortality

This is the report of a working party of the UK Children's Cancer Study Group (UKCCSG) and the Society of British Neurological Surgeons [1]. It was published in 1997 by the RCPCH as a result of the observation that although survival rates for central nervous system (CNS) tumours are comparable with the best in the world, coordination of the services involved has been poor. This has led to parents seeking treatments abroad despite their availability in the UK.

Twenty-five per cent of cancers in children under 16 years of age are tumours of the CNS. This amounts to about 350 cases per year in the UK. Five and 10 year survival rates are about 55 and 50%, respectively, and have not changed much over the last decade compared to haematological malignancies where survival rates have dramatically increased. It is not known whether this is because CNS tumours are inherently resistant to treatment or because treatment quality is suboptimal. It is suspected that there may be scope for significant improvement in survival rates for some CNS tumours. In addition to survival rates, it is important to look at quality of life issues as CNS surgery, chemotherapy and radiotherapy can all leave a child with significant neurological disability.

In the past decade, up to 90% of children with cancer have been registered with the UKCCSG and received care from the network of childhood cancer centres linked with the UKCCSG. However, many children with CNS tumours have not been registered and this suggests that these children are being denied access to specialist cancer services. These specialist cancer services exist within children's departments or hospitals and provide multidisciplinary teams with paediatric and oncological expertise. In addition there has been little inclusion of these children in clinical trials, just 37% of all children with CNS tumours in 1996.

The report remarks that 'until recently there has been a reluctance among neurosurgeons to refer children to their neurosurgical colleagues with a special interest

126

or training in paediatric neurosurgery'. As a result there are few truly experienced paediatric neurosurgeons and referral patterns for further treatment (chemotherapy and radiotherapy) are very variable and may not be to centres with paediatric expertise. The report recommends that for a population of about 2 million there should be at least one neurosurgeon with a commitment to paediatric surgery and another with some experience in the field. The neurosurgical team should be linked to one of the 22 children's cancer centres identified by the UKCCSG.

The Expert Advisory Group on Cancer recommends that cancer services for children and adolescents should be concentrated within designated cancer centres and not cancer units. There is already evidence that treatment in such centres confers a survival advantage.

Children with CNS tumours should be treated within the guidelines set out in clinical service guidelines, including the 'Patients' Charter: Services for Children and Young People 1996' [2] (see also pages 10–11). These specify that the services should provide the following:

- Prompt, accurate diagnosis: urgent referral for neuroimaging should be made as soon as a CNS tumour is suspected and, if confirmed, immediate referral should be made to a paediatric neuro-oncology centre for assessment and treatment planning.
- Clear recommendations for referral to centres with age specific facilities for cancer treatment and neurosurgery.
- Multi-disciplinary assessment and treatment planning: initial assessment should involve paediatric neurosurgeon and/or neurologist, plus paediatric trained oncologist, neuroradiologist and neuropathologist. There should be effective communication within and between all disciplines of the team and also between the primary, secondary and tertiary health teams. There should also be effective communication with the child and their family.
- Treatment and follow up within an age specific environment: in-patient areas should be designed for children and staffed by paediatric trained nurses. Clinical staff should be trained to give chemotherapy safely. Paediatric trained rehabilitation teams should be available. These should be coordinated by a paediatric oncology liaison team. Play leaders should be part of the team. There should be paediatric equipped neurosurgical theatres and intensive care unit available. These should have facilities for controlled hypothermia, intracranial pressure and cerebral function monitoring. There should be special areas for day admissions and routine follow-ups should be kept to a minimum.
- Skilled psychosocial and educational support: staff are required to give diagnoses and explain treatments. They should be trained in breaking bad news. There should be easy access to support from social services and psychologists. Information should be easily accessible. Links with the education system should be maintained and a statement of special education need should be considered where appropriate. Family accommodation should be available.
- Easy access to other specialist facilities: there needs to be high quality palliative care available as 50% of these children die and the remaining 50% may need some palliative care at some point in their treatment. Paediatric community nurses should be involved from the outset. Complementary therapies are increasingly being accepted as useful adjuncts. There should be special arrangements for long term follow up and advice regarding adult issues (e.g., fertility, employment).

- Multi-disciplinary quality assurance, audit, teaching and research: there should be regular team meetings and internal and external audit should be practiced. Registration with the UKCCSG should be ensured and treatment data should also be collected to facilitate research. Where possible, children should be entered into clinical trials.

At the end of the report there are a series of common clinical scenarios. For each of these there is the case history followed by an outline of the approach to management, including a discussion of the pathology, and epidemiology. Most of the case histories are of the presentation of various differing tumours. There is also a case of a child 8 years post-treatment for cerebellar medulloblastoma who has poor growth and disruptive behaviour as a long term sequel of cranio-spinal radiotherapy. Symptoms and signs of intracranial tumours are discussed in terms of their anatomical site and effects, e.g. disturbances in growth and behaviour in midline tumours.

REFERENCES

1. *Guidance for Services for Children and Young People with Brain and Spinal Tumours*. London: Royal College of Paediatrics and Child Health. 1997.
2. NHS. *The Patients' Charter: Services for Children and Young People*. Department of Health. 1996.

Miscellaneous Documents

A Blueprint for Clinical Governance

KEY POINT

- Outlines the RCPCH strategy for clinical governance

Published in 1999, this report sets out the RCPCH strategy for clinical governance [1]. The blueprint consists of the college's aims, and an outline of how it will set, deliver and monitor standards of clinical performance.

The college defines clinical governance as 'promotion of good practice, prevention of poor practice and intervention in failing practice'. The college sets out its wider aims for clinical governance. These entail developing and maintaining the standards of individual members and of child health services as a whole. This also requires identification of poor practice and the support of individuals to improve their practice. The internal structure of the Royal College as it relates to clinical governance is described in terms of the various committees and their roles. Key to this is the Clinical Governance Board which coordinates the actions of the other committees.

The setting of standards is examined. This entails the setting of examinations (DCH and MRCPCH), monitoring of training and continuing professional development. The College will also set guidelines for evidence-based practice.

The College proposes to maintain standards by working with Trusts, postgraduate deans and the Royal Colleges. Key to this is the use of audit and reviews of personal performance. Through continuing professional development individual members can ensure they comply with expected standards, and where necessary improve personal practice.

The monitoring of standards is examined. The College already monitors training and this role is to be extended into service accreditation and performance review. The College will continue to advise on all consultant appointments, to ensure that candidates are suitably experienced and trained for the post.

The GMC will expect regular revalidation of doctors. This is likely to involve peer review, and participation in continuing professional development. The college will detail a list of core competencies which consultants will be expected to have. It is envisaged that the College will arrange retraining for those who do not meet expected standards.

REFERENCE

1. *A Blueprint for Clinical Governance*. London: Royal College of Paediatrics and Child Health. 1999.

British Paediatric Surveillance Unit Annual Report 1998/1999

KEY POINTS

- The BPSU studies the epidemiology of selected uncommon childhood conditions
- About 12 conditions are selected each year
- Monthly surveillance cards sent to paediatric and other consultants
- Provides powerful data corroborated by other sources of information
- Enables guidance of medical practice, rapid response to public health emergencies and service planning

The British Paediatric Surveillance Unit (BPSU) was set up in 1986 by the British Paediatric Association (now the RCPCH) to study the epidemiology of uncommon conditions affecting child health. It is funded partly by the DoH and partly by the research teams using it for their data collection.

Each year up to 12 conditions are chosen and surveillance cards are sent to about 1800 consultants in paediatrics and other relevant specialties, such as pathology, throughout the UK and Republic of Ireland. The conditions chosen are ones which are important to paediatricians and are not so common that the number of notifications exceeds approximately 300 per year. These orange cards need to be filled in monthly. In 1998, 93% of cards were returned completed [1].

When cases are reported the information is sent to the relevant research team. This research team then contacts the consultant for further information as agreed in their protocol by the Ethics Committee. The results of this are reported back to the BPSU along with confirmation of case identification and any duplications.

Since being set up, 40 surveillance projects have been completed. This has provided some very useful evidence with which to guide medical practice (disease prevention and treatment) and service planning. For instance there are enough cases of congenital syphilis, rubella and HIV infections to justify antenatal screening. In addition this monthly reporting allows rapid response to public health emergencies. The BPSU has been so successful that other counties have started to use this type of surveillance and there is now a newly established International Organization of Paediatric Surveillance Units which currently has 10 members. The BPSU recognizes that for various reasons reporting is never 100% but point out that because it validates its data by collaborating with the PHLS, death registration and hospital episode data, the data it does produce is powerful.

The main studies undertaken in 1998 were as follows:

1. Survey of cerebral oedema and death following diabetic ketoacidosis (DKA): preliminary results indicate an incidence of cerebral oedema of 7/1000 cases of

DKA. When it occurs, 25% of children die and 40% are left with significant neurological or neuropsychological disability. Those most at risk are those under 4-years-old and those in whom the diagnosis of diabetes mellitus is new.

2. Congenital Brachial Plexus Palsy: the completed results from this study are not yet available but the incidence was found to be significant at 0.5–1/1000 live births.

3. Congenital Rubella Syndrome: surveillance of congenital rubella syndrome started in 1971 with reporting to the National Congenital Rubella Surveillance Programme.

4. Encephalitis in children aged 2 months to 3 years: this looked particularly at the role of human herpes virus HHV-6 and HHV-7. Results are still being collated.

5. Fatal/severe allergic reactions to food ingestion: this looked at the number of children in whom the reaction was severe enough to be hospitalized and/or who died.

REFERENCE

1. British Paediatric Surveillance Unit (BPSU). *Annual Report 1998/1999*. London: Royal College of Paediatrics and Child Health. 1999.

The Cochrane Library

KEY POINTS

- Electronic publication
- Systematic reviews
- Distillation of the latest evidence on the effects of health care interventions
- Maintained and updated by an international organization: the Cochrane Collaboration
- Aims to help people (including those receiving care) make well-informed decisions about health care

The Cochrane Library is an electronic publication available on CD-ROM (quarterly) and on the Internet. It aims to provide high quality information to support evidence-based practice. The library includes The Cochrane Database of Systematic Reviews (CDSR). Reviews are mainly of randomized controlled trials of the effects of health care. Evidence is included or excluded on the basis of explicit quality criteria to minimize data. Data are often combined statistically, with meta-analysis, to increase the power of the findings of numerous studies, each too small to produce reliable results individually. These reviews are maintained and regularly updated by contributors to the Cochrane Collaboration.

In addition to the CDSR the library includes:

- A Database of Abstracts of Reviews of Effectiveness (DARE): structured abstracts of systematic reviews from around the world, which have been critically reviewed by reviewers at the NHS Centre for Reviews and Dissemination at the University of York.
- The Cochrane Controlled Trials Register (CCTR): bibliographic information on controlled trials.
- Other sources of information on the science of reviewing research and evidence-based health care:
  1. the Cochrane Review Methodology Database (CRMD): a bibliography of articles and books on the science of research synthesis;
  2. a handbook on critical appraisal and the science of reviewing research;
  3. a glossary of methodological terms;
  4. contact details for Collaborative Review Groups and other entities in the Cochrane Collaboration;
  5. 'Netting the Evidence': where to find information on the internet on using evidence in practice.

Topics covered in the systematic reviews are very varied. The following are examples of reviews currently included in the CDSR:

- allergen immunotherapy for asthma;
- antibiotics for sore throat;
- colloid solutions for fluid resuscitation;
- deoxyribonuclease for cystic fibrosis;
- early postnatal (<96 hours) corticosteroids for preventing chronic lung disease in preterm infants;
- elective high frequency jet ventilation versus conventional ventilation for neonatal respiratory distress syndrome in preterm infants;
- interventions for treating headlice;
- repeated lumbar or ventricular puncture to prevent disability or shunt dependence in newborn infants with intraventricular haemorrhage.

REFERENCE

1. The Cochrane Library can be accessed at URL: http://www.cochrane.org

The National Newborn Screening Programme – An Audit of Phenylketonuria and Congenital Hypothyroidism Screening in England and Wales

KEY POINTS

- An audit of PKU and CHT screening in the UK
- Only one audit standard was met: quality assurance
- Identifies delays in laboratories receiving samples and in treatment being started
- Made recommendations to update and improve the screening programme
- Suggests national standards

The Department of Public Health Medicine at United Medical and Dental Schools Guy's and St Thomas's, London published this audit of the newborn screening programme in 1998 [1].

Phenylketonuria (PKU) has been screened for since 1969 and congenital hypothyroidism (CHT) since 1981. This is done by a heel prick blood test at about 1 week of age. In some parts of the country other disorders such as cystic fibrosis and haemoglobinopathies are also screened for. The aim of screening for these conditions is to enable early treatment to prevent the severe consequences of the disease processes [2]. There has been anecdotal evidence over the years that there are certain babies with PKU or CHT who 'slip through the net'. As the number of tests available to screen for other genetic and rare metabolic diseases increases, it is becoming even more important to evaluate the overall performance of the newborn screening programme in the UK [3].

The report starts by defining screening and screening criteria, looking at the Wilson and Jungner criteria of 1968 [4] which include that the condition being screened for should be an important health problem for which there are acceptable, sensitive and specific tests and suitable, available treatments. The whole process should be cost-effective.

The report then describes the UK newborn screening programme. The first stage of the programme involves midwives, health visitors and neonatal nurses informing parents of its existence and then taking the specimens by heel prick at 5–10 days of life. Informed verbal consent to testing should be obtained from the parents.

The laboratories perform the tests and results are reported to other laboratories, child health information departments, midwives or health visitors, hospital paediatricians and GPs. Monitoring of the programme is performed by laboratories, health visitors, community paediatricians, child health information departments, midwives and public health physicians. When a positive test is identified the screening laboratory notifies the Director of Public Health, GP or paediatrician. The paediatrician is then responsible for further testing and treatment. Several registers are used for cross checking results to ensure that infants do not get missed out.

The audit began in 1994 and ran over 2 years. It looked at the newborn screening programme in England and Wales. It was funded by the DoH and was guided by a steering group.

The audit had three main aims:

1. to develop national standards for the programme;
2. to compare practice against standards across England and Wales, and to identify the reasons for the failure to achieve these standards;
3. to identify and encourage implementation of the changes needed to achieve the standards set.

The national standards were drawn up by adapting existing standards which had been developed from local audits and creating an ideal standard. This ideal included that parents should be informed about the programme prior to sampling, and should be given the result when available. Results should be checked against a register for the whole area and when untested infants are identified, they should be tested as soon as possible. All infants who test positive should be seen and treated as soon as possible: 95% within 21 days and 100% within 35 days. There should be individuals responsible for monitoring and coordinating the programme.

A postal survey was performed to compare practice with the ideal standards drawn up. Response rates varied from 74 to 100%. Further interviews were conducted in some areas.

In essence, the audit found that standards were not met. However, most of the outcome and process standards were nearly met.

- 95.8% of notified births were screened by 4 weeks of age (standard = 99.5%);
- 83% of results were available by 20 days after birth (standard = 95%);
- 81% of the untested infants were identified by 28 days (standard = 100%);
- 75% of parents were informed of results;
- 92% of positive cases started on treatment by 21 days, and 99% by 35 days.

The main area of delay was in specimens reaching the laboratories. However, in CHT cases there was often significant delay between infants being seen by paediatricians and the start of treatment. This suggests uncertainty about the management of cases. In general there was a lack of data collection including that on positive cases and follow up, and a lack of service coordination. Communication with parents was also found to be deficient.

The report commented that part of the problem with the UK newborn screening programme is as a result of lack of a strategic overview. It recommends updating of the technology used, clarification of national policy and establishment of a quality assurance programme. It also recommends that the NHS research and development programme funds research looking at screen-detected and missed cases including a review of existing registers.

At the back of the report are some examples of the monitoring schemes in place in some districts and a detailed suggested protocol for performing and monitoring the screening programme.

Re-audit of these standards to complete the audit cycle was anticipated.

REFERENCES

1. Streetly A, Corbett V. *The National Newborn Screening Programme - an Audit of Phenylketonuria and Congenital Hypothyroidism Screening in England and Wales.* London: Department of Public Health Medicine, UMD Guy's and St Thomas's Medical Schools. 1998.
2. Hall DMB. *Health for all Children: Report of the Third Joint Working Party on Child Health Surveillance.* 3rd edn. Oxford: Oxford University Press. 1996.
3. Simpson N, Walker S, Randall R, Lenton S. Audit of Neonatal Screening. *Arch Dis Child* 1997; 77: F228–234.
4. Wilson JMG, Jungner YG. *Principles and Practice of Screening for Disease.* Public Health Papers no 34. Geneva: World Health Organization. 1968.

INDEX

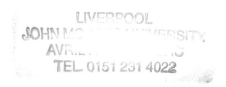